Rheumatic Diseases
An Introduction for Medical Students

T. Gibson, MD, FRCP

*Consultant Physician, Department of Rheumatology,
Guy's Hospital, London*

Butterworths
London Boston Durban Singapore Sydney Toronto Wellington

First published 1986

© Butterworth & Co. (Publishers) Ltd. 1986

British Library Cataloguing in Publication Data

Gibson, T.
  Rheumatic diseases: an introduction for medical students.
  1. Rheumatism
  I. Title
  616.7'23   RC927

ISBN 0-407-00315-0

Library of Congress Cataloging in Publication Data

Gibson, T. (Terence)
  Rheumatic diseases

  Includes bibliographies and index.
  1. Rheumatism.   2. Arthritis.   I. Title
  [DNLM: 1. Arthritis.   2. Rheumatism.   WE 544 G45lr]
  RC927.G53   1986   616.7'23   86-2673
  ISBN 0-407-00315-0

Photoset by Butterworths Litho Preparation Department
Printed in England by Page Bros. Ltd, Norwich, Norfolk

Preface

Rheumatic diseases cause much temporary and permanent disability. At least a quarter of complaints seen by family practitioners are rheumatic in nature. Many doctors experience a sense of inadequacy when confronted with these problems because, until recently, rheumatology was not taught to medical students in a comprehensive fashion. Medical school curricula have adapted slowly to alterations in the patterns of illness and to the changing expectations of patients. There are still schools where the teaching of rheumatology is not given the emphasis it warrants.

This book has been written principally for medical students. Its intention is to provide more information than is available in a general medical text so that those receiving rheumatology tuition may have an easily understandable aid without recourse to a detailed volume for the specialist.

Each subject is presented as it might be on a ward round. The history, clinical findings, differential diagnosis, investigations, pathogenesis and treatment are considered in that order. The emphasis is unashamedly clinical but basic science is not ignored. References are appended to each chapter. These are not comprehensive sources of information but are intended to impart the flavour of recent research and to stimulate further enquiry. It is hoped that the ultimate beneficiaries of the book will be patients with rheumatic diseases.

T. Gibson, MD, FRCP

To Jane

Contents

viii

1
The structure of joints

Three types of joint are found in man. First, fibrous joints, such as those between tibia and fibula which allow little movement. Secondly, cartilaginous joints which occur in the spine, symphysis pubis and at the manubriosternal junction. Their articulating surfaces are covered with hyaline cartilage and separated by fibrocartilage. These allow limited movement but can withstand great pressure. Thirdly, synovial joints which predominate and are mainly peripheral structures that permit a wide range of movement.

Synovial joints

There is a common arrangement of bone, cartilage, synovium and capsule (*Figure 1.1*). Stability is achieved by ligament and muscle attachments. Ligament and cartilage variations are seen as in the knee where there are internal cruciate ligaments and two fibrocartilaginous menisci. Blood vessels enter the joint where the capsule merges with periosteum. Nerve fibres supply the capsule but very few are seen in the synovium.

Normal synovium

This lines the joint capsule and is deflected on to the bone surface to meet the margin of the articulating cartilage. Synovial membrane also lines tendon sheaths and joint bursae. It is normally 1–3 cells thick. The sub-synovial layer is relatively acellular and contains vesels, fibroblasts and connective tissue. Two major types of lining cell can be distinguished by electron microscopy (*Figure 1.1*). Type A cells resemble macrophages and are derived from circulating monocytes. They contain large vacuoles and their membranes form filopodia. Like monocytes, they contain surface

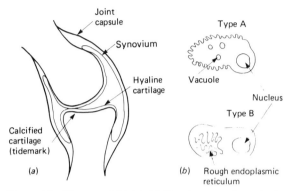

Figure 1.1   The synovial joint. (a) The structure of a typical synovial (diarthrodal) joint. (b) The electron microscopic appearance of Type A and B synovial lining cells

receptors for the Fc chains of immunoglobulins and for complement. They carry HLA DR gene products and one of their immune functions is that of antigen processing and presentation. Type B cells resemble fibroblasts and contain much rough endoplasmic reticulum. In health these constitute two-thirds of the lining cells. They have a secretory role and synthesize hyaluronic acid. This product makes the thin layer of synovial fluid highly viscous, enhancing its lubricating qualities. A small number of cells have Type A and B characteristics and are known as Type C cells.

Normal articular cartilage

The hyaline cartilage forms a smooth, glistening surface over which lies a lubricating film of synovial fluid. It is avascular and contains small numbers of chondrocytes. In adults these cells do not replicate except in disease. Their nutritional requirements are obtained by diffusion from synovial fluid and they produce collagen and proteoglycans. The latter combine with a high water content to form a gelatinous matrix. Cells and matrix are constrained by arching bundles of Type 2 collagen. These extend vertically from the subchondral bone and nearer the surface lie horizontally. Water moves out of cartilage in response to increased pressure, contributing to its buffering effect.

Proteoglycans comprise a protein core to which the glycos-aminoglycans, chondroitin sulphate and keratin sulphate are attached. These are loosely linked by threads of hyaluronic acid to form high molecular weight aggregates. As cartilage ages, the keratin to chondroitin sulphate ratio increases.

Spinal joints

The major joints in the spine are cartilaginous (*Figure 1.2*). The vertebral body end plates comprise thin layers of hyaline cartilage. These are separated by an intervertebral disc which contains a central nucleus pulposus surrounded by a meshwork of Type 1 and Type 2 collagen bundles to form the annulus fibrosus.

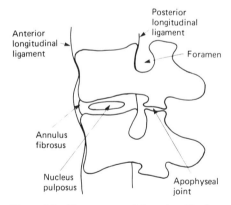

Figure 1.2   The structure of the spine. The intervertebral space is buffered by the disc. The facetal (apophyseal) articulation is a synovial joint. Note the supporting ligaments and the intervertebral foramen through which nerve roots emerge

The nucleus has a high water content and small quantities of Type 2 collagen and proteoglycan. The water and proteoglycan contents of the disc decline with ageing.

The vertebral bodies are also united by four apophyseal or facetal joints, two above and two below. These are synovial joints. In the cervical spine the small uncovertebral joints of Luschka adjoin the discs and some believe that these are also synovial joints. Stability of the spine is aided by the anatomical arrangement of the apophyseal joints and by ligaments. The anterior and posterior longitudinal ligaments extend the length of the spine attached to the vertebral bodies. The anterior ligament is thicker and stronger than the posterior. The laminae are linked by the ligamentum flavum. The sacroiliac joints are part of the axial skeleton. These are synovial joints, differing from peripheral joints only by a parallel arrangement of collagen bundles in the iliac hyaline cartilage.

2
The principles of joint examination

Taking a history

Rheumatic symptoms can never be ignored even when they seem incidental to a patient's main complaint. They must be considered in relation to the history as a whole and never be attributed simply to the effects of ageing.

To help establish a diagnosis and gauge the impact of symptoms on function, a history should attempt to answer the following questions:

1. What are the main joint symptoms – *pain, stiffness* or *swelling*? Are there any accentuating or relieving factors?
2. What *sites* are affected? Are one or more joints involved? Is the spine a source of symptoms? If peripheral joints are affected are these the large joints, the fingers and toes, or both? Is the distribution of affected sites symmetrical?
3. What is the relationship to *time*? Are the symptoms intermittent, migratory or chronic? What is their duration? Was the onset acute or insidious? At what time of day or night are symptoms worse?
4. Are there *extra-articular symptoms* which could be relevant? Has there been fever, weight loss, skin rash, eye inflammation, bowel disturbance, urethritis, Raynaud's phenomenon?
5. Is there a *family history* of joint pain? If so, is it similar to the patient's complaint?
6. What *other illness* has the patient had either currently or in the past? What medication is the patient receiving?
7. How *disabling* are the symptoms? Can the patient work and continue leisure activities? Are washing, bathing, dressing, cooking and shopping difficult or impossible? Does the patient require a walking stick, frame or wheelchair to maintain mobility?

8. What are the patient's *domestic circumstances?* This is crucial information if there is any degree of disability. Does the patient live alone? What assistance is available in the house? Are there any steps or stairs? If disability is severe and of long standing have social services been alerted? Have aids been provided?

The examination

A careful history should direct attention toward the joints involved. The constraints of time may prevent a detailed examination of every joint, but their gross appearance should be noted and no examination of the musculoskeletal system is complete without an assessment of spinal movement.

Just as a history of joint pain needs to be interpreted in the light of other symptoms, so abnormal joint findings need to be evaluated in the context of other abnormalities revealed by a general examination. There are some anatomical areas which are particularly rewarding of careful examination. These are the skin, nails and eyes.

Peripheral joints

There are a number of principles which are applicable to the examination of *all* peripheral joints:

1. *Observe.* Compare with neighbouring or contralateral joints for *swelling, discolouration, deformities* and *muscle wasting.*
2. *Feel* for *warmth* compared with other joints, and for *tenderness* by light pressure. If swelling is present attempt to determine whether this is due to a joint effusion or soft tissue thickening. Effusions are recognized by fluctuance.
3. *Assess movement.* See what a patient can achieve when instructed to move a joint. This is *active* movement. Pain or stiffness may impair voluntary movement so *passive movement* with the examiner gently moving the joint while the patient relaxes may provide a better illustration of restricted motion. Compare the range of movement with a contralateral healthy joint if possible. During movement palpate for crepitus.

Determine whether there is *increased movement* due to ligamentous laxity.

One peripheral joint which is affected by a wide range of disorders is the knee. *Figure 2.1* illustrates the principles of examination applied to this joint. Pain in the knee may be referred from the hip, examination of which is also illustrated (*Figure 2.2*).

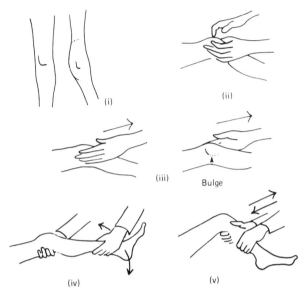

Figure 2.1 Examination of the knee

(a) *Observe:* (i) Compared with the opposite joint there is swelling, muscle wasting and varus deformity of the left knee (varus is inward and valgus is outward pointing deformity). An important aspect of evaluating any joint in the lower limb is an examination of walking and the pattern of gait. Deformities of the knee such as the one illustrated here often become more obvious when the patient stands

(b) *Feel:* The knee is warm. In (ii) the examiner is attempting to detect an effusion by balloting the patella and feeling for transmitted pressure. A small effusion may be confirmed by the 'bulge sign'. This involves massaging one side of the knee, then the other to see if a bulge will appear on the initial side (*see* (iii)). While palpating the knee it is also important to feel the popliteal fossa for the presence of a Baker's cyst, a posterior bulging of the joint cavity

(c) *Movement:* Having assessed active and passive movement, the examiner looks for abnormal movement. In (iv) the knee is held slightly flexed and collateral ligament laxity assessed by lateral movement. In (v) the examiner is looking for antero-posterior instability. Abnormal forward movement, a positive 'anterior draw sign' would indicate laxity or a tear of the anterior cruciate ligament. During the assessment of knee flexion and extension, a hand placed on the patella will indicate the presence of crepitus

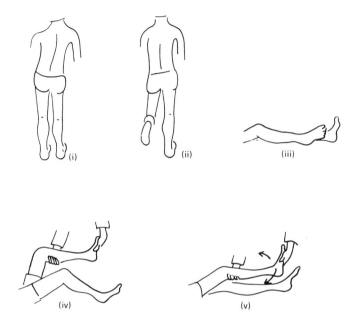

Figure 2.2   Examination of the hip

(a) *Observe:* In (i) the patient has a scoliosis because the pelvis is tilted to the right. Disease of the right hip has caused real shortening of the leg due to bone and cartilage loss. There is also functional shortening due to flexion deformity. This can be confirmed by measuring the leg length. On walking, the patient has a limp. The pelvis falls to the contralateral side when he stands on the involved hip producing a 'Trendelenberg gait' (ii). This is due to weakness of the hip abductors. (iii) shows that the patient has wasting of the quadriceps and holds the leg in flexion and external rotation. These are characteristic deformities of hip disease

(b) *Movement:* On flexing the contralateral hip (iv) the right leg rises off the couch at the extremes of movement. This reflects an inability of the diseased hip to extend. As the pelvis begins to rotate in response to flexion of the normal hip, the abnormal joint is obliged to travel with it. Not only is the hip held in external rotation but internal rotation is severely limited. This is the first movement to be restricted in hip disease. In (v) the examiner is attempting to rotate the hip which is held in flexion. When severe pain is present, rotation is better assessed by rolling the extended leg on the couch. Flexion, abduction and adduction are also evaluated and the range of movement compared with that of the healthy joint

The spine

Examination of the spine involves application of the same general principles:

1. *Observe.* Look for evidence of deformity. In the cervical spine this may take the form of head rotation or tilting (*torticollis*). In the dorsal spine there may be a forward curvature or *kyphosis.* This may be combined with rotation of the spine and deformity of the thorax, so called *kyphoscoliosis.* In the lumbosacral area there may be flattening of the usual hollow of the spine or the natural lordosis. This usually implies muscle *spasm.* Sideways curvature of the spine denotes *scoliosis.* If scoliosis is present it may be functional, due to protective muscle spasm, or structural due to congenital deformity. It may also result from disparity of leg lengths. If scoliosis disappears on sitting it is unlikely to be due to a structural abnormality. With the patient standing, a comparison of the level of the gluteal folds and the popliteal creases behind the knees may indicate differences of leg length.
2. *Movement.* Restricted flexion, extension, lateral flexion or rotation of the spine may affect isolated segments. A crude notion of what constitutes a normal range of movement may be easily obtained by the examiner studying his own spine. Forward flexion must be assessed by observing the dorsal and lumbar regions and not the hands as they attempt to touch the floor. Much flexion takes place at the hips and an observer may be easily deceived by a patient with a rigid spine whose ability to touch the floor with finger tips is unimpaired. Placing two fingers on different vertebral spines may give some idea of whether the vertebral bodies move on one another during flexion. This may be given more precision by marking two points on the spine and measuring their separation on flexion. A more formal approach for the lumbar spine is the modified Schober index. This is obtained by marking a point on the lumbar spine at the level of the dimples of Venus and then one point 10 cm above and another 5 cm below. The separation of the distal points beyond 15 cm gives some measurement of lumbar spine flexion.
3. *Feel.* The cervical spine may be palpated for *tenderness* with the patient seated but areas of dorsal and lumbosacral tenderness are best determined with the patient lying prone. It is common to find tenderness of paravertebral muscles, the buttocks and sacroiliac joints even when the source of symptoms

lies within the spine itself. Such referred areas of tenderness can be confusing. Various techniques have been described for determining tenderness of the sacroiliac joints. These include pressing on the sacrum with the patient prone, pressing on the ilium with the patient lying sideways and forced flexion and adduction of each hip with the patient supine. None is better than palpating directly over the sacroiliac joints.

4. *The extremities.* Comparing *leg lengths* is an integral aspect of lumbar spine examination. This is simply achieved by measuring the distance between each anterior superior iliac spine and medial malleolus.

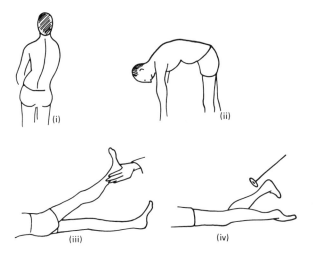

Figure 2.3   Examination of the lower spine

(a) *Observe:* The patient in (i) has a scoliosis concave to the right. The buttock folds and knee creases are level but measurement of leg lengths is necessary to rule out the possibility that the scoliosis is due to shortening of a leg

(b) *Movement:* In (ii) forward flexion of the lumbosacral spine is seen to be restricted. Other movement may also be impaired. A cursory inspection suggests that forward flexion is near normal because the patient can almost touch the floor. However, it is quite clear that the lumbar spine remains rigid and flexion is occurring mainly at the hips. Finger tips or marks placed over two lumbar spinal processes would confirm lack of movement at this level

(c) *Feel:* Tenderness may be apparent

(d) *Extremities:* Straight leg raising is restricted on the right side (iii). The femoral nerve stretch test is negative. A neurological examination reveals an absent right ankle jerk (iv) indicative of S1 nerve root compression. The clinical picture is consistent with a lumbar disc protrusion

With the patient supine, straight leg raising can be assessed. In health, the leg can be flexed to 90 degrees and beyond. When nerve roots supplying the sciatic nerve are compressed, straight leg raising will be limited. Some individuals have taut hamstring muscles which impair movement so a comparison of each leg is important in order to ascertain the significance of any restriction. The reproduction of pain or paraesthesiae by straight leg raising is further evidence of neurological involvement. The test can be embellished by forcefully dorsiflexing each foot with the leg raised as high as possible. This extra stretching of the sciatic nerve may induce pain not previously apparent. This is the sciatic nerve stretch test. An analogous test of nerve roots supplying the femoral nerve, the femoral nerve stretch test, may be performed by flexing the knee with the patient lying prone. Pain in the back or thigh during this test may indicate upper lumbar nerve root compression.

Examination of the spine is concluded by a search for neurological abnormalities of the upper or lower limbs. Wasting, weakness, diminished reflexes or sensory impairment may help to define the precise level of a nerve root lesion.

Some important aspects of lumbar spine examination are shown in the illustrated example of *Figure 2.3*.

Recording the findings

There are no conventional ways of documenting clinical abnormalities of the joints. This poses difficulties for the accurate follow-up of diseases which are so often chronic. Recording the distribution of involvement is essential, and to facilitate this many specialist units utilize an illustration of the human form on which the areas of disease may be mapped. A descriptive account is adequate.

Recording the severity of change is the principal difficulty. Muscle wasting and joint swelling can be estimated by measuring limb girth and joint circumference using defined anatomical landmarks. Deformities and joint movement may be assessed using a goniometer (*Figure 2.4(b)*). This is practicable only for large joints and requires anatomical precision. The range of movement may be expressed in degrees, e.g. 0/90 or 20/140. The top figure represents the resting joint angle and would exceed zero if there were some angulation due to deformity. This really encompasses a way of expressing both the extent of deformity and the range of movement.

Tenderness is worth noting. It may be the only expression of joint disease. Some observers simply note the number of tender joints but this approach can be made more sensitive by constructing a tenderness score in response to light pressure or joint rotation (0 = none, 1 = slight, 2 = patient winces, 3 = patient

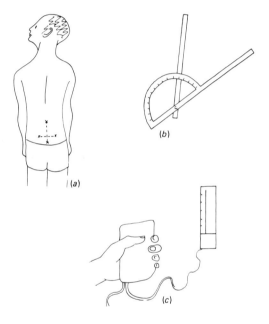

Figure 2.4   Methods of measurement in rheumatology. (a) Spinal flexion. The spine has been marked over the dimples of Venus, lines drawn between them and another extending 10 cm above and 5 cm below. The distance moved between the ends of the vertical line can be used to gauge the extent that the lumbar spine moves on forward flexion. (b) A goniometer which can be used to measure the range of joint movement in one plane. (c) An inflated bag of special design attached to a sphygmomanometer. This can be used to record grip strength

withdraws). A composite score can be derived which relates to the activity and progression of chronic polyarticular diseases.

For disorders affecting the small joints of the hands, grip strength is another semi-quantitative method of assessing severity. This is achieved by using a special cuff attached to a sphygmomanometer inflated to 30 mmHg (*Figure 2.4 (c)*). An ordinary cuff rolled tightly is a less satisfactory alternative. The best or average of three recordings for each hand is then documented.

Spinal disease can be evaluated best by measuring the range of movement and straight leg raising. A goniometer may be utilized for recording cervical rotation and flexion as well as straight leg raising. The modified Schober Index is the most useful means of evaluating lumbar spine flexion (*Figure 2.4(a)*). Measurements of extension and lateral flexion are possible but more difficult to standardize.

In addition to these, the duration of morning stiffness is often a helpful guide to disease severity. Pain and stiffness may also be recorded on a visual analogue scale but this approach is more appropriate to research than ordinary clinical practice.

More important to the patient is functional ability. Observers should make every attempt to assess changes in the degree of disability by asking the questions outlined in the section devoted to history.

Sequential notes incorporating the measurements outlined above are mandatory for charting the progress of patients with chronic rheumatic diseases. Clincial impressions are often misleading and inadequate.

Further reading

FRIES, J. (1983). Toward an understanding of patient outcome measurement. *Arthritis Rheum.*, **26,** 697

HUSKISSON, E. (1974). Measurement of pain. *Lancet,* **2,** 1127

MACRAE, I. and WRIGHT, V. (1969). Measurement of back movement. *Ann. Rheum. Dis.*, **28,** 584

MALLYA, R. *et al.* (1982). Correlation of clinical parameters of disease activity in rheumatoid arthritis with serum concentration of C reactive protein and ESR. *J. Rheum.*, **9,** 224

3
Mechanisms of inflammation

Acute and chronic inflammation contribute to the pathology of most joint diseases. In many instances the initiating event is unknown but much has been learned about the mechanisms involved. The precise role and relationship of many of the factors discussed are not clear, but the immune system and its humoral products are crucial elements in this process.

Cellular components of inflammation

Macrophages

These are derived from circulating monocytes and are distributed widely in the body, including the joints. They possess receptors for C3 and the Fc portion of immunoglobulin, and these facilitate the phagocytosis of foreign antigens. They also secrete a wide range of products including the protease enzymes collagenase, β-glucuronidase and elastase. Other secreted factors include prostaglandin E_2, oxygen metabolites and complement.

The surface of macrophages possess HLA DR gene products. These are involved in the immune recognition and processing of antigen by the macrophage (antigen presentation). This step is crucial to the stimulation of lymphocytes by another macrophage product, interleukin-1 (Il-1). This peptide also induces synovial cells to secrete prostaglandin E_2 and collagenase, the liver to release the acute phase reactant, C reactive protein (CRP) and chondrocytes to secrete proteases. Il-1 is also produced by cells other than macrophages and has a more extensive range of effects.

14

Lymphocytes

Three major types of lymphocyte can be recognized. T cells are the most numerous and are differentiated in the thymus. They are distinguished by the presence of surface receptors for sheep erythrocytes. B cells mature in the marrow and lymphatic system and are recognized by the presence of surface immunoglobulins. A smaller population of cells do not exhibit the surface properties of T or B cells and are called null lymphocytes.

Antigenically distinct subclasses of T cells reflect the wide range of T cell activities. Helper T cells in close proximity to antigen presenting macrophages secreting interleukin-1 (Il-1) respond by secreting interleukin-2 (Il-2). This initiates T cell proliferation amongst those cell subsets which are reactive to the antigen (*Figure 3.1*). Proliferating helper cells may be further involved in the stimulation of B cells to produce immunoglobulins.

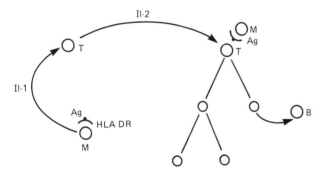

Figure 3.1 Macrophage and lymphocyte interactions. M = macrophage; T = T lymphocyte; B = B lymphocyte; Ag = antigen; HLA DR = HLA DR products on a macrophage; Il-1 = interleukin-1; Il-2 = interleukin-2

A second subset, suppressor T cells, functions in opposition to helper cells. Modulation is achieved by opposing effects on B cell activity and by subtle interactions between them. A third subset, cytotoxic T cells, is important in the destruction of foreign cells. Null cells are also cytotoxic both in the presence of antibody (antibody-dependent cellular cytotoxicity–ADCC) and in its absence (natural killer activity–NK activity). Null cells are also stimulated by interleukin-2 and interferon, the latter produced by T cells and fibroblasts.

Immunogenetics

The immune system, functioning as it does to defend the host against foreign antigens, must recognize self as well as the nature and functions of cells involved in immune responses. The genes whose products are important for immune function are collectively known as the major histocompatibility complex (MHC). They are found on the short arm of chromosome 6 and include the human leukocyte antigens (HLA) which are expressed on the membrane of most nucleated cells (*Figure 3.2*). The sequence of several genes within the MHC has been determined and each HLA site or locus has been designated with the letter A, B, C or D.

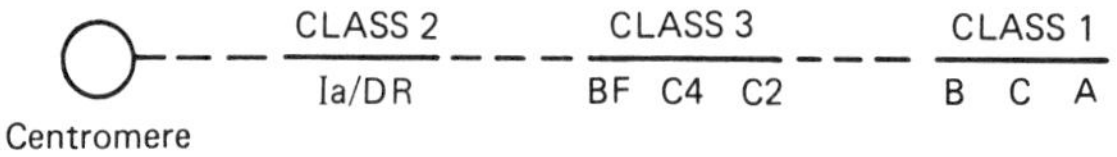

```
O - - - CLASS 2 - - - - - CLASS 3 - - - - - CLASS 1
            Ia/DR           BF  C4  C2          B  C  A
Centromere
```

Figure 3.2 MHC genes and their distribution on chromosome 6. These are only a few of the MHC genes

Genes within the MHC also code for the complement components C2, C4 and Factor B (BF). Inheritance of MHC genes is characterized by a tendency for the genes from each parent to be transmitted together without breakage. Each gene sequence from a single parent represents a haplotype and both haplotypes combine to form the genotype, i.e. each parent contributes one of several possible genes (alleles) to each locus. The full sequence of paired alleles is referred to as the phenotype, e.g. HLA-A1, A4; B7, B27, etc.

The HLA ABC genes are called class 1 genes. These are involved in T lymphocyte recognition. Class 2 genes are represented by HLA Ia/DR and these are associated with regulation of antibodies through T helper and suppressor lymphocyte functions. The Class 3 genes are important for the production of complement components.

Granulocytes

In most rheumatic diseases the polymorphonuclear leukocyte plays an important role, but the other granulocytes, the eosinophils, basophils and mast cells (the tissue counterparts of basophils) may also be implicated.

The accumulation of polymorphs is a uniform characteristic of inflammation. These are attracted to sites of tissue damage by any of several chemotactic factors. The complement derivatives C5a and C3b are the most important but products of arachidonic acid, lymphocytes, mast cells, macrophages, platelets and polymorphs themselves may all exhibit chemotactic properties. Eosinophils, basophils and circulating macrophages may also be attracted by some of these factors, but eosinophils are especially responsive to the chemotactic factor of anaphylaxis (ECF-A), produced by mast cells in response to IgE.

Polymorphs ingest and degrade particulate material. This process is enhanced by coating (opsonization) of particles with IgG or the C3b component of complement.

The following phagocytic sequence is shared by mononuclear macrophages. Adherence of material (e.g. bacteria, immune complexes, debris or crystals) is followed by a burst of oxygen consumption associated with increase of the hexose monophosphate shunt. Oxygen is converted to superoxide, hydrogen peroxide and hydroxyl free radicals. Phagocytosis is achieved by infolding of the polymorph membrane to achieve a phagosome. This migrates centrally, fusing with a lysosomal granule and its contents. Lysosomal protease enzymes digest the engulfed material. During this process oxygen products and proteases are also secreted into the exterior.

Platelets

Activation of platelets leads to their aggregation and release of serotonin (5-hydroxytryptamine), prostaglandins and small quantities of hydrolytic and proteinase enzymes. These changes may be induced directly by collagen, thrombin, immune complexes, complement components, crystals and platelet activating factor (PAF) derived principally from basophils and mast cells.

Humoral components of inflammation

Complement proteins

Inflammatory mechanisms are, to a large extent, dependent on this complicated system and its diverse actions. Complement proteins circulate as inactive precursors. The first components to be recognized have the prefix C and are numbered in the order they were first identified. These constitute the classical pathway which is activated by IgM or IgG containing immune complexes (*Figure 3.3*). The first component (C1) contains three sub-units, C1q, C1r

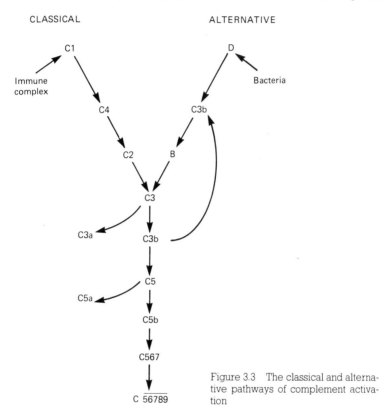

Figure 3.3   The classical and alternative pathways of complement activation

and C1s. C1q binds to the Fc fragment of immunoglobulin, thereby initiating conversion of C1 to an active protease C̄1. The cascade of activation which follows involves cleavage of complement precursors to form further proteases, the enzymatic activity of which is indicated by a bar over the number. The second component of the pathway is C4 which is cleaved by C̄1 to form a new enzyme C̄1̄4̄. An inhibitor in serum, C1 esterase inhibitor, may prevent this sequence. Other inhibitors may influence later aspects of the cascade. The action of C̄1̄4̄ on C2 produces C̄4̄2̄ which cleaves C3. Cleavage products arising at each step are designated a, b, c or d. Thus, the larger product of C3 is termed

C3b which in the presence of C$\overline{42}$ cleaves C5 to C5a and C5b. The interaction C5b with C6, 7, 8 and 9 without their cleavage produces an enzyme which is capable of disrupting cell membranes. Micro-organisms may activate complement by a slower and alternative pathway involving two factors designated B and D (*Figure 3.3*). In this latter cascade, C3 is cleaved by the enzyme C3bBb.

The terminal sequence is the same as in the classical pathway. The most important activities of complement are listed in *Table 3.1*.

TABLE 3.1 Activities of some of the more important complement components

C1q	Aggregation of immune complexes
C2 products	Increases vascular permeability
C3a	Stimulates release of serotonin from platelets, histamine from basophils and mast cells
C3b	Opsonization prior to phagocytosis by polymorphs and macrophages which have C3b surface receptors
C5a	Chemotactic factor for polymorphs and macrophages

Immunoglobulins

Immunoglobulins are a family of structurally similar proteins whose variable amino acid arrangement provides an infinite variety of antibodies against foreign antigens. They are secreted by stimulated B cells (plasma cells) each of which can synthesize only one type of immunoglobulin at a time.

Each immunoglobulin molecule comprises two light and two heavy polypeptide chains (*Figure 3.4(a)*) Disulphide bridges link segments within each chain and the chains themselves. At one end of the molecule, the N terminus, both heavy and light chains display amino acid variations which contribute to antibody specificity (idiotype). The other end of the molecule, the C terminus, shows some variability but is relatively constant. The segments of light and heavy chains bearing the N terminus are known as the Fab fragment (fragment antigen binding). The remainder of the molecule ending at the C terminus is the Fc fragment (fragment crystallizable). Each Fab segment carries two antigen combining sites. The Fc portion of the molecule is involved in binding of the antibody to cells such as macrophages and in the activation of complement.

Two types of light chain occur, kappa (κ) and lambda (λ). More than half the light chains are of the κ type. There are five major forms of heavy chain and these differences are reflected in the five major classes of immunoglobulin (Ig): G, A, M, D, and E.

In the circulation IgG is the most abundant. IgA is found predominantly on seromucous surfaces. Heterogeneity of the heavy chains results in four subclasses of IgG and two of IgA. The initial antibacterial antibody response is effected by IgM. This comprises five molecules linked by a polypeptide chain (J chain) to produce a pentameric macroglobulin bearing ten antigen binding sites (*Figure 3.4(b)*). It is a highly effective agglutinator.

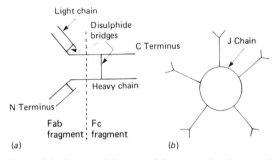

Figure 3.4   Immunoglobulins. (a) Structure of an immunoglobulin molecule. The N terminus is sometimes called the variable (V) region and has many possible amino acid sequences in contrast to the C terminus, the constant region, which has only one sequence for each class of immunoglobulin. The chains are linked by disulphide bridges. (b) The pentameric structure of IgM. The J chain is a non-immunoglobulin linking five identical subunits by a series of disulphide bridges (not indicated)

IgM and IgD appear on the surface of lymphocytes. The antibody present in the least quantity is IgE. It attaches to basophils and mast cells and its serum level increases during parasitic infections. Unlike IgG and IgM, both IgA and IgE activate complement via the alternative pathway.

Rheumatoid factors

Antibodies which react with the Fc portion of IgG are termed rheumatoid factors (RF). These may be of any immunoglobulin class including IgG itself. The classic rheumatoid factor of rheumatoid arthritis is an IgM antibody. The exceptional agglutinating qualities of this immunoglobulin allow relatively easy recognition of IgMRF. Sheep red cells or other particles coated with aggregated animal IgG and exposed to human serum will agglutinate in the presence of IgMRF. The role of rheumatoid factors in joint diseases is unknown. IgMRF can activate complement and precipitate soluble immune complexes. Low titres may be detected in elderly subjects, in bacterial endocarditis and infectious tropical diseases. Larger amounts are characteristic of rheumatoid arthritis and other connective tissue diseases.

Immune complexes

Antigen–antibody complexes may form in the circulation or locally in tissues. Usually, but not exclusively, the antibody is IgG. Immune complexes circulate in health and their formation accelerates removal of foreign antigen. Large molecules, with an extensive lattice between antigens and antibodies, are removed quickly by phagocytic cells. Large complexes are likely to form in situations where antigen and antibody are present in high but unequal concentrations. They are capable of causing tissue damage and may precipitate on blood vessel walls if their removal is impaired by reticuloendothelial saturation. Precipitation is associated with activation of complement and the induction of inflammation. Immune complexes demonstrate a predeliction for vessels of the glomerulus, joints and skin.

Immune complexes may be measured by several techniques which do not always produce concordant results. Estimation of the quantity which binds to a specific amount of radiolabelled C1q resembles the physiological response and is a popular assay.

Cryoglobulins are immunoglobulins which precipitate in the cold. Mixed cryoglobulins are immune complexes containing more than one immunoglobulin class and these invariably display RF activity. They arise in connective tissue diseases as well as in a wide range of infections. Unmixed cryoglobulins contain only one class of immunoglobulin and are associated with diseases of monoclonal overproduction, e.g. myeloma.

Antinuclear antibodies (ANA)

These are frequent accompaniments of connective tissue diseases. Some may participate in tissue damage by involvement in immune complexes. In general their pathogenetic significance is unknown. Several methods have been devised for their detection. The lupus erythematosus (LE) cell test, in which nuclear material released from damaged cells is ingested by polymorphs in the presence of antibody, has been superseded by indirect immunofluorescent techniques. In the latter, animal tissue cell smears are incubated with human serum and immunofluorescent labelled anti-human gamma globulin. Serum containing one or more antibodies against antigens of cell nucleus, cytoplasm or membrane will attach to the animal substrate along with immunofluorescent labelled antibody. Both the LE cell and the ANA screening tests are thus capable of detecting several antibodies. Their specificity may be indicated by the pattern of immunofluorescent staining, e.g. anti-histones with rim or homogeneous staining, anti-RNP with a speckled pattern.

Newer methods have allowed identification of antibodies with greater precision. Antibodies against double stranded DNA may be detected by incubation of serum with radiolabelled pure DNA obtained from micro-organisms. Precipitation of formed anti DNA–DNA complexes with ammonium sulphate allows an estimate of the amount of bound DNA (Farr technique). An alternative method employs indirect immunofluorescent staining of the flagellate, *Crithidia luciliae*. This organism possesses a kinetoplast which is rich in double stranded DNA. Antibodies against double stranded DNA are more specific for systemic lupus erythematosus (SLE). Antibodies to single stranded DNA and histones may be detected by other techniques. Histones are basic proteins which combine with DNA, and antibodies against them are characteristic of drug-induced SLE. Another group of antibodies are directed against antigens which can be extracted from animal thymus and are soluble in normal saline (extractable nuclear antigens). These are generally detected by the method of counter-immunoelectrophoresis and they are of interest because some display disease associations which have diagnostic implications. The antigens have been designated Sm, RNP, Ro, La, Jo-1, Pm-Scl, Scl-70 and centromere. Antibodies against RNP are seen in SLE and in all cases of mixed connective tissue disease. Anti-Ro and anti-La occur most frequently in primary Sjögren's syndrome, anti-Jo-1 in polymyositis, Scl-70 in scleroderma and anti-centromere in the variety of scleroderma associated with sclerodactyly, Raynaud's phenomenon and calcinosis.

Prostaglandins

Prostaglandins, thromboxanes and leukotrienes comprise a large and heterogeneous group of low molecular weight compounds which mediate inflammation (*Figure 3.5*). Activation of a cell membrane phospholipase liberates the polyunsaturated fatty acid, arachidonic acid, from the membrane. This is converted by lipoxygenase and cyclo-oxygenase pathways into a cascade of products, some of which exert an important influence on

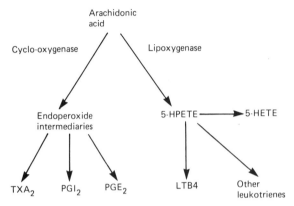

Figure 3.5 The arachidonic acid cascade. TXA2 = thromboxane; PGI_2 = prostacyclin; LTB4 = leukotriene B4

inflammation. These are all rapidly inactivated in the circulation and tissues. PGE_1, PGE_2 and PGI_2 (prostacyclin) cause vasodilatation, thromboxane A_2 induces platelet aggregation and vasoconstriction and is antagonized by prostacyclin. HETE and LTB4 (leukotriene B4) are chemotactic for polymorphs, supplementing the effects of complement component C5a.

Other humoral mediators

Histamine is produced by mast cells and basophils in response to IgE. This has diverse effects and acts on two tissue receptor sites, H_1 and H_2. Its ability to increase vascular permeability may involve both receptors. It may also influence polymorph and lymphocyte function.

Serotonin (5-hydroxytryptamine) is taken up and released by platelets. Like histamine it is an amine and is thought to have a similar effect on vessel walls.

Bradykinin is a kinin which is able to produce vasodilatation as well as increasing vascular permeability. Kallikrein, which acts on kininogen to produce bradykinin, is chemotactic for polymorphs and monocytes. Both kinins are products of the intrinsic clotting system.

Acute phase proteins comprise several proteins whose serum concentrations alter dramatically in response to tissue injury or inflammation. Their role in inflammation is not understood. The best known of these is C reactive protein (CRP). This is produced in the liver in response to interleukin-1. It activates complement and there is some evidence that it may modulate inflammation. Serum amyloid A is a similar acute phase reactant and like CRP its concentration may increase many times following tissue injury. Haptoglobin, fibrinogen and α_1-antitrypsin are other reactants which exhibit modest elevation but pre-albumin is an acute phase protein whose concentration falls during inflammation.

Further reading

DAYER, J. (1985). Mononuclear cell factor–interleukin-1 in rheumatoid arthritis. *Br. J. Rheum.*, **24** (*Supplement 1*), 15

DUKE, O. *et al.* (1982). An immunohistological analysis of lymphocyte subpopulations and their microenvironment in the synovial membranes of patients with rheumatoid arthritis using monoclonal antibodies. *Clin. Exp. Immunol.*, **49**, 22

HUGHES, G. (1984). Autoantibodies in lupus and its variants: experience in 1000 patients. *Br. Med. J.*, **289**, 339

LESSARD, J. *et al.* (1983). Relationship between the articular manifestations of rheumatoid arthritis and circulating immune complexes by three methods and specific classes of rheumatoid factors. *J. Rheum.*, **10**, 411

SPILBERG, I. *et al.* (1982). Induction of a chemotactic factor from human neutrophils by diverse crystals. *J. Lab. Clin. Med.*, **100**, 399

STOBO, J. (1982). The influence of immune response genes on the expression of disease. *J. Lab. Clin. Med.*, **100**, 822

WERNICK, R. *et al.* (1985). IgG and IgM rheumatoid factor synthesis in rheumatoid synovial membrane cultures. *Arthritis Rheum.*, **28**, 742

WILKINS, J. *et al.* (1984). Generation of interleukin-2 dependent T cell lines from synovial fluids in rheumatoid arthritis. *Clin. Exp. Immunol.*, **58**, 1

4
Osteoarthritis

Osteoarthritis (degenerative joint disease; OA) is the most common form of arthritis. The radiological features associated with OA increase in frequency with age but may not be accompanied by symptoms.

Symptoms

Pain, stiffness and swelling are the main complaints. The onset is insidious but trauma may accentuate pain, suggesting an acute arthritis. There may be a past history of injury or disease affecting the involved joint or adjacent bone. Pain is usually confined to one or a few joints and may be worse at the end of the day and after exercise. Nocturnal pain denotes severe disease. Stiffness is less severe than in rheumatoid arthritis (RA), but, as in RA, may be evident after inactivity.

Functional disability reflects the distribution and severity of involvement. Walking, coping with steps and standing from a sitting position are problematic for those with hip or knee disease. Gripping and fine finger movements are impaired when thumb or fingers are involved.

Signs

Although symptoms are usually limited in distribution there may be evidence of generalized osteoarthritis. Heberden and Bouchard nodes situated at the distal and proximal interphalangeal joints characterize hypertrophic generalized OA, a pattern of arthritis which has a familial association and affects women more than men (*Figure 4.1*). The nodes are usually painless or only slightly tender. A pattern of generalized OA may occur in the absence of Heberden nodes but this is less common. Joint swelling caused by osteophytes or effusions, deformities due to cartilage loss or capsular laxity, muscle wasting, tenderness, warmth, crepitus and restricted movement are all variable findings.

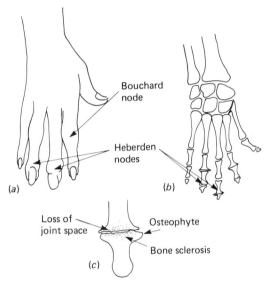

Figure 4.1 Hypertrophic osteoarthritis. (a) Clinical appearance of the hand. (b) Radiological appearance of Heberden and Bouchard nodes. Note also the involvement of the carpometacarpal joint of the thumb. (c) The radiographic appearance of a Heberden node in more detail

The most common example of OA is hallux rigidus. This is usually preceded by chronic valgus deformity of the first metatarsophalangeal joint and is seen more frequently in women. Involvement of the first carpometacarpal joint is almost as common. In the latter condition the thumb is unable to abduct and there is usually thenar muscle wasting. Wrist and shoulder involvement are uncommon but OA of the elbow is seen among men who have engaged in heavy work and is often painless, a reduced range of elbow extension being the only clinical manifestation. Hip disease is usually unilateral and affects women more than men. Pain may be referred to the knee so hip examination is important in all cases of knee pain. Impairment of internal rotation is the first indication of hip disease. Lack of extension and flexion deformity result in apparent leg shortening but true shortening may be caused by loss of cartilage and bone. Both may result in pelvic tilting and compensatory spinal scoliosis. Weakness of the hip abductor muscles results in a Trendelenberg gait. Osteoarthritis of the knee may be associated with flexion, valgus or varus deformities. Crepitus may be pronounced with patellofemoral involvement. Shortening of a leg due to hip disease may induce or accelerate osteoarthritis in the contralateral knee (long leg arthropathy). Osteoarthritis of the ankles is rare except in those with a history of repeated trauma, e.g. footballers.

Differential diagnosis

An insidious onset of pain affecting a single joint in an elderly person is likely to indicate osteoarthrits. Systemic features are absent. Generalized OA may occasionally be confused with rheumatoid arthritis, especially when Bouchard nodes are inflamed. Heberden nodes sometimes become red and tender, resembling gout or psoriatic arthropathy. Presence of a joint effusion and associated warmth at any other involved site may also suggest an inflammatory disorder. It must not be forgotten that occasionally OA coincides with an inflammatory disease. Hip and spinal pain may co-exist because of the mechanical strains imposed on the spine by leg shortening. Determining which is the predominant source of pain may be difficult but is important during assessment for hip surgery.

Investigation

In the absence of coincidental illness, laboratory features of inflammation such as anaemia, high ESR or CRP are absent. The radiological features of OA in order of progression are:

1. loss of joint space;
2. osteophytes;
3. sclerosis of subchondral bone;
4. subchondral cysts;
5. collapse of bone and subluxation.

Minor joint narrowing, sclerosis and osteophytes occur increasingly with age, especially in the spine. Such changes are frequently asymptomatic. Joint effusions should always be aspirated even in the presence of radiological evidence of OA. Examination may reveal unsuspected inflammatory features or crystals. In OA the synovial fluid is viscous and clear or only slightly turbid. The white cell count is usually less than $2.0 \times 10^9 \, \ell^{-1}$.

Aetiology

Osteoarthritis represents the common end-stage of many heterogeneous conditions. The underlying defect of primary generalized OA both with and without Heberden nodes is unknown. There is no obvious predisposing cause in many instances of OA. Subjects with hypertrophic OA of the hands are more likely to develop OA at other sites. Hip involvement in such patients is more likely to be associated with concentric loss of cartilage rather than loss of the superior weight bearing surface which is more common (*Figure 4.2*).

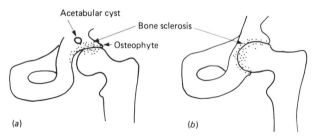

Figure 4.2 Two radiological patterns of OA affecting the hip. (a) The more common picture with loss of the superior weight bearing surface. (b) Uniform loss of cartilage. The latter is characteristically seen in association with Heberden nodes but is also the appearance of hip involvement in inflammatory joint diseases

Predisposing causes include repetitive occupational trauma, fractures affecting articular surfaces or the alignment of long bones, sepsis and chronic inflammatory joint diseases.

Calcium hydroxyapatite crystals have been isolated from OA synovial fluid but their relevance is unclear. Paget's disease, avascular necrosis and epiphyseal dysplasia are other causes. Hip OA may follow congenital hip dysplasia or dislocation. Knee disease may result from disparity of leg lengths or meniscal tears. Acromegaly, diabetes, haemochromatosis, and alkaptonuria (ochronosis) are endocrine or metabolic causes. There may be an association with obesity.

Pathology

At an early stage of OA the cartilage loses its gloss and becomes pitted and fibrillated. In time it may completely disappear to expose underlying bone. Microscopically the initial changes are focal with fibrillation occurring in all planes. The chondrocytes respond by dividing and increasing their activity and size. They tend to congregate in clumps (clones) but as the disease progresses they diminish in number. Vertical fibrillation may form clefts which extend into the bone, and synovial fluid forced along

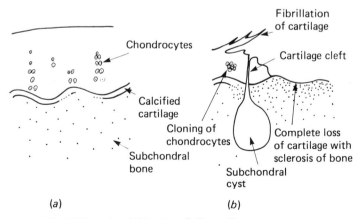

Figure 4.3   (a) Normal and (b) osteoarthritic cartilage

these channels helps to create subchondral cysts which may later collapse (*Figure 4.3*). Structural change is preceded by chemical alterations. The water content of cartilage increases and initially the ratio of chondroitin to keratin sulphate increases. Later, both glycosaminoglycans decline in concentration and the proteoglycan aggregates are disrupted. Subchondral bone becomes thickened and its surface area expanded by the outgrowth of osteophytes.

The joint capsule and ligaments may be stretched by joint effusions and the synovium may become more vascular and oedematous. The subsynovium is infiltrated with variable numbers of perivascular lymphocytes and the synovial lining becomes hyperplastic. The appearance of the synovium may be indistinguishable from inflammatory joint diseases including RA.

These inflammatory changes result in increased exudation of synovial fluid. Unlike inflammatory joint disease, the fluid contains only small numbers of leukocytes and these are usually mononuclear. It is possible that the inflammatory changes contribute to the destruction of cartilage by inducing the release of proteinases from synovium, synovial fluid cells or chondrocytes themselves.

Treatment

Medical

General measures include reassurance, weight reducing diets and modification of activities so that involved joints are not over used. In lower limb disease, quadriceps strengthening exercises, correction of leg shortening with a shoe raise and provision of a walking stick may all be helpful. Physical treatments which provide warmth, e.g. short-wave diathermy, may reduce pain for a few days. Analgesia is better achieved by a regular simple analgesic or non-steroidal anti-inflammatory drug (*see* Chapter 19). Intra-articular corticosteroids may lessen pain for several weeks but should not be repeated more than two or three times. Involvement of the thumb may be treated with an immobilizing splint. A hinged splint is occasionally of value for unstable OA of the knee when surgery is not possible.

Surgical

Surgical fusion of the first carpometacarpal and first metatarso-phalangeal joints may abolish pain. Knee involvement with varus or valgus deformity and preservation of some joint space may benefit from corrections of the deformity by tibial osteotomy. The management of hip and knee OA has been transformed by joint replacement surgery. These are the procedures of choice if pain is severe and disabling.

Course

Radiological progression is not predictable. Hip and knee OA may deteriorate quickly but at other sites the disease may remain unaltered for years. Symptoms may fluctuate in the absence of further changes to the joint and spontaneous but temporary improvement is common. Some believe that radiological deterioration of hip OA may be accelerated by use of non-steroidal anti-inflammatory drugs.

Further reading

BUCHANAN, W. and PARK, W. (1983). Primary generalised osteoarthritis – definition and uniformity *J. Rheum.*, **10,** 4

HOUGH, A. (1983). Variants of osteoarthritis – a pathological overview. *J. Rheum.*, **10,** 2

TESHIMA, R. *et al.* (1983). Comparative rates of proteoglycan synthesis and size of proteoglycans in normal and osteoarthritic chondrocytes. *Arthritis Rheum.*, **26,** 1225

5
Rheumatoid arthritis

This is the most common inflammatory joint disease and is the one most often associated with severe physical handicap. It is three times more common amongst females than males. It may be associated with several extra-articular features and for this reason it is sometimes called rheumatoid disease.

Symptoms

At the outset pain, swelling and stiffness affect joints in succession, becoming established at several sites within months. In the elderly the onset may be associated with sudden involvement of many joints. Another presentation is that of palindromic rheumatism in which the more typical picture of RA is preceded by intermittent episodes of arthritis which may occur over many months or even years. Stiffness tends to be severe and most evident in the mornings.

Some patients attribute the disease onset to physical or psychological trauma or an infectious episode, but there is no good evidence that such factors are of true aetiological significance.

Characteristically, the disease affects the small joints of the hands and feet, especially the second and third metacarpo-phalangeal (MCP), proximal interphalangeal (PIP) and metatarso-phalangeal (MTP). Metatarsal pain may be the initial complaint and may be described as like walking barefoot on pebbles. Large joints may be prominently involved at an early stage. The shoulders seem particularly vulnerable in the elderly. Cervical spine involvement may cause headaches as well as neck pain.

Many simple day-to-day functions such as dressing, bathing and use of the lavatory may be impaired. In severe disease the struggle to perform mundane tasks contributes to fatigue and leads to frustration and depression.

Extra-articular features usually follow the arthritis but weight loss, malaise and fatigue may precede joint symptoms. Nocturnal pain or tingling of the fingers due to carpal tunnel syndrome commonly accompany the earliest symptoms. Olecranon bursitis, subcutaneous nodules, dependent oedema and tenosynovitis may also be early manifestations. Rarely, exertional dyspnoea due to rheumatoid lung disease or symptoms of other extra-articular features may occur before joint involvement is apparent.

Signs

Joints

There is usually a striking symmetry of swelling and tenderness of metacarpophalangeal, proximal interphalangeal and other joints (*Figure 5.1*). In established disease there may be ulnar drift of the fingers, subluxation of the metacarpophalangeal joints and boutonnière or swan-neck deformities. Tenderness of the distal interphalangeal joints may be present but swelling is rare. Finger flexion may be limited by small joint swelling and inflammation of the flexor tendon sheaths. The latter may temporarily obstruct extension of fingers from a position of flexion (triggering).

Swelling of the wrists may be difficult to distinguish from that of the overlying extensor tendon sheaths. It is at this site that tendons are most prone to rupture because of inflammatory damage. This event may be first recognized by sudden inability to extend a finger.

Elbow swelling is usually confined to fullness of the space between the olecranon and radial head. Extension of the joint may be severely impaired.

Painful restriction of the shoulders is common and is a severe handicap. Overlying muscles may disguise joint swelling. Painful chewing and local tenderness may denote temporo-mandibular involvement.

Impaired and painful head rotation indicates cervical spine inflammation. The neck region is the only area of the spine which is

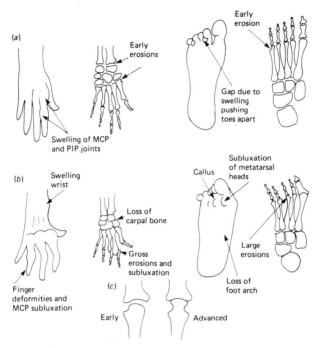

Figure 5.1   The clincial and radiographical appearance of the hands and feet in rheumatoid arthritis; (a) early, (b) advanced, and (c) closer view of early and advanced erosions

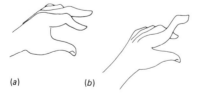

Figure 5.2   Typical rheumatoid hand deformities; (a) boutonnière, and (b) swan-neck

affected in RA and this occasionally causes neurological complications.

Hip involvement is not usually seen in early disease but must be suspected when pain occurs in the groin, buttock or in an apparently normal knee. The signs are identical to those of osteoarthritis of the hip and restriction of internal rotation is the first abnormal sign. Any swelling of the joint is obscured by surrounding tissues.

As at other sites knee swelling may be due to synovial thickening or effusion. A small effusion may be demonstrated by the bulge sign and larger quantities by the patella tap test. Valgus or varus deformities and collateral or cruciate ligament laxity may occur. Baker's cysts are common and these may leak to produce ankle oedema or may rupture and cause painful swelling of the calf and foot, simulating a deep vein thrombosis.

Tenderness, swelling and restriction of ankle, sub-talar and mid-tarsal joints tend to occur later in the disease. It may be difficult to determine clinically which of these joints is the worst affected. Loss of foot arches and valgus deformity of the ankle contribute to deformity and pain (*Figure 5.3*). Valgus deformities of the ankles often coincide with similar deformities of the knees.

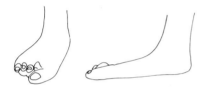

Figure 5.3   Late rheumatoid deformities of the foot with valgus of the ankle and big toe, clawing of the second toe and flattening of the longitudinal foot arch

In the forefeet the brunt is borne by the metatarsophalangeal joints. Downward subluxation of the metatarsal heads results in overlying callus formation with pronounced tenderness (*Figure 5.1(b)*). There is usually little obvious swelling of the toe joints but puffiness over the dorsal aspect of the metatarsals and of the interphalangeal joints may be seen.

Inflammation of a single joint which is disproportionate to other evidence of disease activity suggests the possibility of septic arthritis. This complication is usually caused by *Staphylococcus aureus* in the presence of an infectious focus such as leg ulceration.

Extra-articular features

These are nearly always seen in seropositive patients with high titres of IgM rheumatoid factor.

Skin

Nodules are virtually exclusive to patients with positive rheumatoid factor tests and are seen most commonly on the elbows and ulnar borders of the forearms (*Figure 5.4(a)*). They may occur at other sites subjected to pressure including the Achilles tendons, buttocks, occiputs and fingers.

Palmar and peri-ungual erythema occur in 30%. The cause is unknown. Cutaneous vasculitis may be manifest by small, brown, nail fold infarcts and skin ulceration (*Figure 5.4(b)* and *(c)*). The

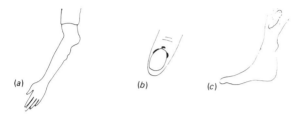

Figure 5.4   Extra-articular features of RA. (a) Subcutaneous nodules and olecranon bursitis; (b) nail fold infarcts; and (c) a nodule in the Achilles tendon and leg ulceration

latter usually arise on the legs but can occur at any site exposed to pressure. They may resemble venous stasis ulceration and can extend rapidly, becoming secondarily infected.

Eyes

Dryness of the eyes, mouth and other mucosal surfaces are features of Sjögren's syndrome. Eye inflammation may take the form of episcleritis or scleritis. Rarely, the cornea and sclera may undergo deep ulceration (scleromalacia). This complication is more common in the presence of Sjögren's syndrome. Blue sclera are common in long-standing RA due to increased scleral transparency through which the pigmented choroid becomes visible.

Lungs

Cigarette smokers are more susceptible to pulmonary complications (*Figure 5.5*). Fibrosing alveolitis may result in finger clubbing, cyanosis and crackles at the lung bases. Pleuritic pain may be associated with a rub or signs of pleural effusion.

Radiology may reveal rheumatoid nodules in the lung parenchyma but these are not necessarily associated with clinical signs.

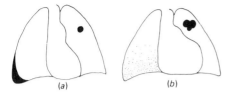

Figure 5.5 Chest radiographs in RA. (a) Pleural effusion and a solitary nodule; (b) fibrosing alveolitis, enlarged heart due to pericardial effusion and the appearance of Caplan's syndrome

Wheezing due to chronic airways obstruction and coarse crackles due to bronchiectasis may also be more common in RA.

Heart

Pericarditis is known to occur in 30% but in general this is a subclinical phenomenon. A rub may occasionally be heard. Constrictive pericarditis is a rare complication but must be considered when signs of right heart failure appear resistant to treatment. Conduction defects and valve dysfunction are also rare features and are caused by rheumatoid granulomata developing within the myocardium.

Nervous system

A mild sensory peripheral neuropathy sometimes accompanies nail fold infarcts and other evidence of cutaneous vasculitis. Mononeuritis multiplex is a manifestation of severe vasculitis and has been associated with increased mortality.

Cervical spine involvement predisposes to forward subluxation of the atlas or of other vertebral bodies (*Figure 5.6*). Such changes

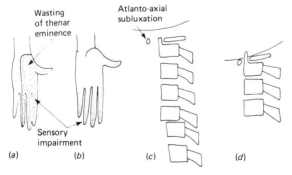

Figure 5.6 Neurological complications of RA. (a) Carpal tunnel syndrome; (b) peripheral neuropathy; (c) atlanto–axial and C5-6 subluxation; (d) upward subluxation of the odontoid peg into the foramen magnum

may be apparent in almost 40% of long-standing cases but less than 2% develop cervical cord compression. Less frequently, destruction of the atlas allows upward subluxation of the odontoid peg to cause medullary cord compression (*Figure 5.6(d)*).
Patients with cord compression may complain only of weakness and tingling of the arms. The distribution of sensory impairment may resemble that of a peripheral neuropathy but increased muscle tone, accentuated reflexes or an extensor plantar response should suggest the correct diagnosis.

Muscles

Disuse wasting of the small muscles of the hands, quadriceps and other sites is usual. Proximal weakness and wasting may be due to a specific myopathy but florid muscle inflammation (polymyositis) is not a feature.

Bone

Diffuse osteoporosis may occur and fractures of long bones may result.

Felty's syndrome

The concurrence of RA, splenomegaly and neutropenia occurs in about 1% of hospital patients with RA. Patients may experience recurrent and sometimes severe infections. Other clinical features may include leg ulceration, skin pigmentation, lymph node enlargement and hepatomegaly. Active synovitis may be minimal but joint deformities are usual. Occasionally, Felty's syndrome may precede evidence of arthritis. Nodules, high titres of IgM rheumatoid factor and a positive test for ANF in 90% are characteristic findings. The neutropenia may be associated with anaemia and thrombocytopenia. The neutropenia appears to be largely due to increased peripheral destruction of polymorphs containing immune complexes.

Oedema

Dependent oedema in RA may be caused by inflammation of ankle and foot joints, immobility, pressure on veins due to prolonged sitting, leakage of a Baker's cyst, fluid retention caused by anti-inflammatory drugs or a combination of these. Deep vein thrombosis is rare in RA, even during prolonged bed rest. Heart failure or other incidental causes may need to be considered and constrictive pericarditis must not be overlooked.

Nephrotic syndrome requires early exclusion by examination for proteinuria. This complication may be secondary to treatment with sodium aurothiomalate or D-penicillamine. In the absence of such a cause, amyloid nephropathy is the most likely explanation and this may be confirmed by rectal or renal biopsy. Amyloid may be deposited at other sites such as liver and spleen. In this pattern of systemic amyloidosis a glycoprotein called amyloid P component (AP) is found in association with fibrillar chains of amyloid A (AA). The latter resembles serum amyloid A (SAA), an acute phase protein which is elevated in RA. This protein may be the source of amyloid A. There is no effective treatment for amyloidosis in RA beyond control of arthritis. Renal amyloid is frequently fatal.

Differential diagnosis

Clinical distinction from other causes of chronic polyarthritis is usually easy if there is symmetrical involvement, rheumatoid nodules or other characteristic extra-articular features. Olecranon and Achilles tendon swelling due to gouty tophi or xanthomata may resemble rheumatoid nodules and occasionally cause confusion.

Psoriatic arthropathy and Reiter's syndrome tend to be associated with an asymmetrical arthritis, ankylosing spondylitis and other spondylarthropathies with predominantly large joint involvement and crystal-induced synovitis is characteristically an acute mono-arthritis. RA presenting with inflammation of one or more large joints or as palindromic rheumatism may be difficult to distinguish from these disorders.

Investigations

Haematology

The erythrocyte sedimentation rate (ESR) is usually elevated and is an excellent index of disease activity.

Hypochromic anaemia is common and also reflects disease activity. The red cells resemble those of iron deficiency anaemia and because serum iron is reduced in active RA, distinction can be difficult. Serum iron binding capacity is often equivocal and since serum ferritin behaves as an acute phase protein in RA it is an unreliable indicator of true iron deficiency. Iron deficiency occurs frequently because of the effect of anti-inflammatory drugs on the gastric mucosa. Its presence can be confirmed only by bone marrow examination or the response to oral iron. In the anaemia of active RA bone marrow iron stores are normal or increased.

The absolute and relative numbers of leukocytes are often normal but there may be a lymphopenia.

The platelet count is increased in active RA and this tends to parallel other laboratory indices of inflammation.

Serology

A positive Rose Waaler or RA latex test for IgM rheumatoid factor (RF) is found in 70%. It has been argued that some or all of the patients who never exhibit abnormal titres of IgM RF have a different disease. 10% of RA patients have a positive test for ANF.

Serum complement levels are normal except in severe vasculitis. Immune complexes as measured by $C1q$ binding or other tests are usually elevated.

C reactive protein (CRP) is an acute phase reactant which fluctuates with the degree of joint inflammation. Some prefer to use CRP rather than ESR as a monitor of activity.

Biochemistry

Mild liver dysfunction often accompanies early disease. Renal function is normal except when impaired by anti-inflammatory drugs or amyloidosis.

Serum immunoglobulins are diffusely elevated.

Radiology

Views of the hands and feet are helpful in establishing diagnosis and following the progression of the arthritis. The metatarso-phalangeal joints are often the first sites to be affected by erosions which may occur in the absence of symptoms. In the hands, the ulnar styloids, metacarpophalangeal and proximal interphalangeal joints may all exhibit marginal erosions at an early stage (*see Figure 5.1*). Involved joints may be associated with progressive bone erosion, loss of cartilage, juxta-articular osteoporosis and subchondral cysts. Ankylosis may also occur especially at the wrists where fusion may be associated with complete loss of one or more carpals (*see Figure 5.1(b)*). Seronegative RA patients may be particularly prone to such wrist involvment. Osteoporosis may be generalized affecting the spine and long bones.

Abnormalities of the sacroiliac, dorsal and lumbosacral spine do not occur but in the neck there may be loss of disc space, ankylosis of vertebral bodies and laminae or subluxation. Extension and flexion views are necessary to determine the presence and extent of vertebral slip. Subluxation occurs most often at the atlanto-axial joint where destruction of the ligament between the odontoid and anterior arch of the atlas may be associated with erosion of the odontoid (*see Figure 5.6*). Normally, forward movement at this site does not exceed 2mm. Radiographs of the cervical spine are important for RA patients undergoing surgery because anaesthetic procedures may inadvertently cause spinal cord damage if subluxation is unrecognized.

A chest film is a mandatory investigation of arthritis and in RA may yield evidence of pleural effusion, fibrosing alveolitis or nodules. Solitary nodules require biopsy to exclude incidental pathology. Patients exposed to silica dusts, as in coal mining, may develop multiple nodules in the lung parenchyma (Caplan's syndrome). These may coalesce or cavitate. The pleural effusions of RA are characteristically exudates with low glucose levels.

Aetiology

The cause of RA is unknown. It has a worldwide distribution and is more common in females. In Caucasians susceptibility is increased by possession of HLA DR4. This occurs in 60% of RA patients and 15% of healthy subjects. Its presence in RA is associated with IgM RF and more severe disease.

Infections have long been suspected as a precipitating cause. At various times mycoplasmas, diphtheroids, Epstein-Barr virus and other micro-organisms have been implicated but none has been proven to be relevant.

Pathogenesis

A wide range of immunological and biochemical mechanisms is involved in the pathogenesis of RA. The initiating event is unknown although it is presumed that the immune responses in RA are directed at foreign or altered antigen. The importance of HLA DR gene products in the reaction between macrophages and lymphocytes may indicate a genetically predetermined response to one or more antigens.

The crucial role of lymphocytes in the evolution of the arthritis can be judged by their presence in rheumatoid synovium and the beneficial response to their therapeutic suppression or removal.

Activated lymphocytes in synovial tissue, lymph nodes and spleen produce increased quantities of immunoglobulins, some of which act as rheumatoid factors. In seronegative RA only IgG and IgA RF can be detected. It is not clear whether RFs play a causal role or are simply instrumental in clearing harmful material by the reticuloendothelial system. Both IgM RF and the immune complexes formed by RFs and IgG have the potential for perpetuating inflammation by activating complement. Some patients exhibit antibodies against type II collagen, the significance of which is unclear.

Paradoxically, lymphocytes involved in cell-mediated immunity tend to be hypoactive in RA. Their responsiveness *in vitro* may be improved by interleukin-2 (Il-2), suggesting that lymphocytes in RA may produce deficient amounts of this lymphokine. These observations and the hyperactivity displayed by B cells point to some disorder of suppressor and helper T cell interactions. Antibody-dependent cytotoxicity (ADCC), a function performed by null lymphocytes, may also be defective.

The different pathways which may be involved as part of the inflammatory response (*see* Chapter 3) may all contribute to the persistent synovitis of RA and its extra-articular features.

Pathology

In the early stages of joint inflammation there is increased vascularity of the subsynovium and a superficial infiltration by polymorphs.

The vascular engorgement is associated with increased production of synovial fluid. Initially, small numbers of mononuclear cells are found in the joint cavity but polymorphs are eventually attracted in large numbers and become the predominant synovial fluid cell.

In contrast to the synovial fluid, lymphocytes (mainly T cells) accumulate in the subsynovium. These may have a perivascular distribution and occasionally resemble lymphoid follicles. Rarely, rheumatoid nodules arise within the synovium. Immunoglobulins, rheumatoid factors and immune complexes are formed within the joint cavity where they are ingested by polymorphs, macrophages and synovial lining cells. This sequence, together with the stimulatory effect of interleukins, may account for the potentially harmful liberation of the degrading enzymes cathepsin D, elastase, collagenase, hyaluronidase, β-glycosaminodase, β-glucuronidase and free oxygen radicals from synovial fluid polymorphs and monocytes, synovial lining cells and cartilage chondrocytes. These may all have a detrimental effect on cartilage but it is not clear to what extent their actions are dissipated by the presence of natural inhibitors.

Persistent synovial inflammation may result in a marked increase of synovial bulk. The lining layer increases from a few to several cells thick and type A cells may increase disproportionately. There may be marked villous formation with surface fibrin formation. Lining cells are shed into the synovial fluid.

The hypertrophied synovium encroaches over the articular cartilage to form pannus. The margin of the pannus contains macrophages, fibroblasts and mast cells and invades cartilage and subchondral bone (*Figure 5.7*). These erosive changes initially

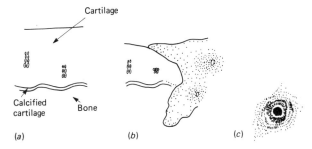

Figure 5.7 Histopathology of RA. (a) Normal cartilage. (b) Pannus eroding cartilage and bone. Note the perivascular collection of chronic inflammatory cells. (c) A rheumatoid nodule with fibroblasts arranged like fencing (palisades) around a central necrotic area

develop at the margin of joints where the protective cartilage is thinnest.

The joint may lose the stabilizing influence of the capsule and ligaments as these become distended by effusion or synovial swelling. Joint laxity and a diminished synovial fluid viscosity may accelerate cartilage degeneration by imposing mechanical stresses and by reducing the efficient lubrication of the articulating surfaces.

Bone adjacent to the joints becomes porotic although the sclerosis of secondary osteoarthritis may follow as inflammation regresses. The erosions may undermine cartilage, coalesce to form cysts and lead to collapse of the subchondral bone. There may be bone resorption, ankylosis or both.

Rheumatoid nodules are the only diagnostic pathological feature of RA. They comprise a central necrotic area surrounded by orderly layers of fibroblasts arranged like fencing (palisades). Other chronic inflammatory cells may also be apparent (*Figure 5.7*).

Rheumatoid vasculitis affects medium or small vessels and is associated with fibrinoid necrosis of the media and thrombus in the lumen. It is likely that these lesions are due to immune complex deposition in the vessel wall and may be associated with reduced serum complement levels. A more benign vasculopathy is caused by intimal thickening of digital vessels.

Treatment

General

Rest is an important but occasionally neglected aspect of treatment. Patients who believe that they will become immobile if they do not exercise vigorously need to be educated in the value of rest. This may be achieved by sitting or lying quietly for a defined period or by bed rest in hospital if joint inflammation is severe, loss of independence threatened or social circumstances prevent proper provision of care.

Rest of individual joints can be achieved by splints worn at night or throughout the day by those confined to bed. Working wrist splints may immobilize painful wrists but allow use of the fingers.

Exercise is of some value in maintaining morale and muscle bulk. The help of physiotherapists is invaluable in encouraging the use of muscles without stressing inflamed joints.

During periods of uncontrolled synovitis or where joint damage has resulted in permanent disability, there is some risk of dietary deficiency, especially amongst those living alone. Expert dietary advice may be helpful.

Most RA patients develop a degree of physical handicap, at least temporarily. The provision of aids such as modified door handles and eating utensils can help sustain independence. Occupational therapists are trained to determine the need and best application of these aids and the requirement for wheelchairs, ramps, bath seats, hand rails and structural alterations to the home (*see* Chapter 20). For the most severely disabled, social support in the form of district nurse, meals on wheels and other voluntary agencies may need to be mobilized.

Medical

First-line

Pain is the symptom from which patients demand most relief. This may be partially achieved by a regular anti-inflammatory agent supplemented by simple analgesics. These measures also reduce joint stiffness and improve functional capacity.

Salicylates remain the anti-inflammatory drugs against which the effects of all other products are measured. These need to be given in a relatively high dosage to produce a demonstrable anti-inflammatory effect. For this reason soluble aspirin is not the best choice because at this dose gastrointestinal side effects are common. Other salicylate preparations such as aloxiprin lessen this risk but many other drugs have been developed as substitutes (*see* Chapter 19). Indomethacin, naproxen and ibuprofen are examples, but no anti-inflammatory preparation is entirely devoid of gastrointestinal side effects and none has a better anti-inflammatory effect than large doses of salicylate.

Simple analgesics which have no anti-inflammatory action include paracetamol, paracetamol-dextropropoxyphene and codeine. These are of value as supplements to anti-inflammatory drugs but do not by themselves provide ideal treatment.

Intra-articular corticosteroid injections of long-acting preparations such as methyl prednisolone or triamcinolone may be very helpful in reducing inflammation of single joints. Large joints such as the knee and wrist are more suitable for injection than small joints (*Figure 5.8*). Prior local anaesthetic is unnecessary except when the techniques are being learned. Pain induced by the irritant effect of steroid crystals may be lessened by adding local anaesthetic to the injected material. Absorption of steroid from the joint may have a transient systemic effect. Injection of single joints should not be repeated more than two or three times in a year because of the risk of accelerated cartilage destruction.

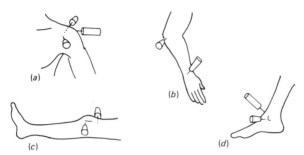

Figure 5.8   Common intra-articular injection techniques. (a) Anterior and posterior approach to the gleno-humeral joint and laterally to the sub-acromial space; (b) elbow via pouch formed between olecranon and radio-humeral articulation, and dorsum of wrist; (c) medial approach to knee with needle placed beneath the patella and laterally into suprapatellar space; and (d) anterior and medial approaches to ankle joint

The above drugs are used to control symptoms and do not have any effect on ESR, rheumatoid factor or the progression of the disease.

Second-line

Patients with obviously severe disease as manifest by early functional impairment, florid synovitis, high titres of rheumatoid factor, extra-articular features or early radiological evidence of joint damage require more than non-steroidal anti-inflammatory drugs. Less severe cases with unremitting activity over a period of several months also require second-line therapy.

The therapeutic choices for second-line treatment are limited and carry a high risk of toxicity (*Table 5.1*). For this reason and because some patients with RA pursue a mild course without disability it is prudent to monitor each patient's progress closely, introducing second-line treatment only when justified by the clinical situation.

Sodium aurothiomalate is given as a weekly injection until either substantial improvement is observed or the cumulative dose has

TABLE 5.1 Second-line drugs

Drug	Dose	Main side effects
Sodium aurothiomalate	50 mg i.m. weekly until remission or 1.0 g then 50 mg monthly	Rash, proteinuria, bone marrow suppression, stomatitis, mouth ulcers, metallic taste
D-penicillamine	125 mg daily for one month increasing by 125 mg every month to maximum of 1.0 g daily	Loss of taste, rash, proteinuria, thrombocytopenia, bone marrow suppression, myasthenia gravis
(a) Chloroquine (b) Hydroxy-chloroquine	(a) 200 mg daily (b) 200–400 mg daily	Rash, headache, corneal and retinal deposition
Azathioprine	50–150 mg daily	Gastrointestinal, liver dysfunction, rash, bone marrow suppression
Sulphasalazine	0.5 g initially increasing by 0.5 g weekly to 2.0–3.0 g daily	Dyspepsia, nausea, rash
Dapsone	50–100 mg daily	Haemolytic anaemia, nausea, bone marrow suppression
Prednisolone	2.5–20 mg daily	Obesity, thin skin, osteoporosis, diabetes, hypertension, atheroma, hair loss, fluid retention, adrenal suppression
Cyclophosphamide	50–100 mg daily	Bone marrow suppression, haemorrhagic cystitis
Methotrexate	10–25 mg weekly	Gastrointestinal, bone marrow suppression, liver and renal dysfunction

reached 1.0 g. Maintenance injections are then continued indefinitely at monthly or more frequent intervals. An oral gold preparation (auranofin) has been developed but this is probably not so effective as the injectable preparation and is associated with more gastrointestinal disturbance.

D-penicillamine is prescribed initially in a small dose, increasing by small increments at monthly intervals to lessen the risk of toxicity. The final dose is the lowest necessary to sustain improvement without causing side effects.

Sodium aurothiomalate and D-penicillamine have similar therapeutic and toxic effects. Unlike anti-inflammatory drugs they do not have an immediate action on inflammation and improvement may be maximal after 2–3 months treatment or longer. They can reduce ESR, CRP and rheumatoid factor titres and can probably slow disease progression. Their side effects demand that the blood and urine of treated patients should be monitored regularly.

The antimalarials, chloroquine and hydroxychloroquine, have a similar delayed effect on RA but are probably less effective at suppressing disease activity. Corneal deposition is reversible but retinal changes are not and may cause blindness if allowed to progress. This risk is remote with low dosage over 1–2 years but expert eye examination at six-monthly intervals is wise. A reduction of visual fields or clear evidence of retinal deposition should bring treatment to a halt.

Other second-line drugs include the cytotoxic agents azathioprine, cyclophosphamide and methotrexate. Azathioprine is relatively safe and exerts an effect which is equivalent to chrysotherapy (sodium aurothiomalate). These should not be used in young people nor in women of childbearing age. Theoretically they can enhance the risk of malignant disease.

Dapsone may be another preparation with second-line properties but its use is restricted by adverse effects.

Sulphasalazine was introduced many years ago as a treatment for RA. It was abandoned but has been restored as a useful second-line agent.

Corticosteroids have a definite role to play but are best reserved for patients who have not been controlled by aurothiomalate, D-penicillamine, antimalarials or azathioprine, or who have severe extra-articular features. The dose should be as low as possible. The long-term side effects can be debilitating and once corticosteroid treatment has been initiated it is often difficult to discontinue.

Large doses of intravenous steroids or cyclophosphamide may be useful in containing vasculitis. Plasmapheresis and lymphocytapheresis are of no lasting benefit. Lymph node irradiation is an experimental approach which may be of benefit for patients with severe unremitting disease.

Surgical

Several procedures are regularly required in RA. These are:

1. tendon repair;
2. synovectomy;
3. osteotomy;
4. joint replacement
5. arthrodesis

The extensor tendons of the wrist are those which most often require repair. Synovectomy of the wrist is sometimes combined with this procedure but synovectomy is most often performed on knees and elbows. The popularity of small joint synovectomy has declined in Britain. Removal of the inflamed tissue may have long-lasting benefits. Radioactive yttrium and other isotopes have been injected into joints where they may effect medical synovectomy.

Osteotomy of the femur or tibia may help to realign the long bones where normal stress has been disturbed by knee deformity. This may relieve pain and delay the need for arthroplasty.

Joint replacement of hips, knees, shoulders, elbows and MCP joints are all feasible. Arthroplasty has been most successfully applied to weight bearing joints (*Figure 5.9*).

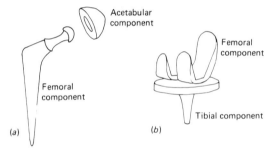

Figure 5.9 Joint prosthesis: (a) hip, (b) knee. The acetabular and tibial components of the hip and knee joints are made of ultra-high molecular weight polyethylene and the femoral components are of stainless steel or a cobalt, chromium and molybdenum alloy. Each section is fixed to bone using acrylic cement

Arthrodesis is a salvage procedure which by fusing joint surfaces may eliminate pain. This is a useful procedure at the wrist but less so when applied to the ankle, hind foot or other joints. Subluxation of cervical vertebrae causing cord compression can be treated by wiring and arthrodesis of one vertebra to another or of the atlas to the occiput.

Course

About one-third of patients have a mild illness with a high rate of remission. Another third progress slowly with minor functional disability. The remainder have more aggressive disease with periods of partial or only brief remission. Such patients may have to abandon work and rely increasingly on a spouse or outside assistance. Those with severe arthritis are more likely to develop extra-articular manifestations. High titres of IgM RF are usually found in these patients but there are exceptions.

Life expectancy is slightly decreased in RA. Infection is a common cause of early death and this risk is increased by corticosteroid treatment. Septic arthritis is a complication which may follow bacteraemia and if this goes unrecognized the risk of death is high. Amyloid nephropathy is another complication which contributes to mortality.

It is thought that the ultimate outlook has been improved by the early and judicious use of second-line treatments but there is no firm evidence to support this. The management of RA is still in a state of imperfection.

Further reading

DAVIDSON, A. *et al.* (1984). Red cell ferritin content: a re-evaluation of indices for iron deficiency in the anaemia of rheumatoid arthritis. *Br. Med. J.,* **289,** 648

EDITORIAL (1984). The viral aetiology of rheumatoid arthritis. *Lancet,* **1,** 772

ELSON, C. *et al.* (1985). Complement activating properties of complexes containing rheumatoid factor in the synovial fluid and sera from patients with rheumatoid arthritis. *Clin. Exp. Immunol.,* **59,** 285

HYLAND, R. *et al.* (1983). A systemic controlled study of pulmonary abnormalities in rheumatoid arthritis. *J. Rheum.,* **10,** 395

IANUZZI, L. *et al.* (1983). Does drug therapy slow radiographic deterioration in rheumatoid arthritis? *New Engl. J. Med.,* **309,** 1023

LUUKKAINEN, R. *et al.* (1983). Relationship between clinical synovitis and radiological destruction in rheumatoid arthritis. *Clin. Rheum.,* **2,** 223

McCONKEY, B. (1982). Rheumatoid cervical myelopathy. *Br. Med. J.,* **284,** 1731

MUTRU, O. *et al.* (1985). Ten year mortality and causes of death in patients with rheumatoid arthritis. *Br. Med. J.,* **290,** 1797

PULLAR, T. *et al.* (1985). Second line therapy in rheumatoid arthritis – a four year prospective study. *Clin. Rheum.,* **4,** 133

6
Spinal pain

Most people experience low back pain or neck ache at some time in their lives and such symptoms could well be considered part of the human condition. Low back pain accounts for more absence from work in Britain than industrial action. Occasionally, spinal pain is caused by serious underlying diseases.

Neck pain

Symptoms

Neck strain

Pain often begins abruptly and may be associated with trauma or sleeping with the head in an awkward position. Such symptoms usually resolve over several days and do not always require medical attention. Whiplash injuries represent one form of neck strain which can take several months to improve.

Cervical disc prolapse

Symptoms are usually acute in onset and are more severe than those of neck strain. Pain may be referred into the scapula, shoulder or hand and there may be associated numbness or paraesthesiae.

Cervical spondylosis

This is a clinical syndrome of chronic or intermittent neck pain, sometimes beginning suddenly but more often insidiously, with

51

referral into the arm, shoulder, occipital or frontal areas. There may be intermittent sensory disturbance or weakness of a hand or arm, dizziness on head rotation and sleep disturbance. Weakness of the legs or bladder disturbance suggest cervical cord compression.

Signs

Neck pain is invariably associated with restricted head rotation. There may be marked muscle spasm with tilting or rotation of the head (torticollis), tenderness of the cervical vertebrae and of the attached muscles.

Where cervical nerve roots have been compressed by disc protrusion or osteophytes, neurological signs will be apparent. Most often there is sensory impairment in the C6, 7, 8 root distributions. There may be weakness of deltoid, biceps, triceps, wrist dorsiflexors or grip. In cervical spondylosis, where root pressure is sustained, there may be associated wasting of these muscles or of the hand (T1). Diminished or absent biceps (C5), triceps (C6) or supinator (C7) reflexes may be found. A brisk finger jerk, increased reflexes in the legs, an extensor plantar response, widespread sensory impairment or a positive Lhermitte's sign (abnormal arm or trunk sensation on head flexion) are confirmation of cord compression.

Cervical spondylosis may occasionally be associated with nystagmus and other abnormal cerebellar signs due to obstruction of vertebral artery blood flow by osteophytes.

Differential diagnosis

Pain in the neck may be referred from the heart or oesophagus although the converse is more frequent with neck symptoms referred to other sites.

Discomfort in the shoulder region is a common accompaniment of neck disorders and may simulate rotator cuff inflammation or adhesive capsulitis. Neck disease may predispose to these conditions which are characterized by painful and restricted shoulder movement.

Referred pain in the forearm requires distinction from lateral and medial epicondylitis. Head and forearm pain or paraesthesiae due to carpal tunnel syndrome or ulnar nerve lesions may cause confusion. Cervical ribs are another but rare cause of arm symptoms.

Polymyalgia rheumatica causes pain and pronounced stiffness of the neck, shoulders and usually of the pelvic girdle. A very high ESR should suggest this possibility. Pancoast tumours may cause shoulder and neck pain as well as neurological symptoms and signs. Metastatic tumours involving the skeleton may also cause neck pain.

Infections of the discs and vertebral bodies are not common. *Staphylococcus aureus* is the most frequent organism in the indigenous British population, but amongst Asian immigrants tuberculosis is a more likely cause of vertebral osteomyelitis. Visitors to countries where unpasteurized dairy products are ingested may be exposed to brucellosis, which is another cause of chronic spinal infection.

Non-infectious inflammatory diseases of the spine such as ankylosing spondylitis and RA should be recognized by their concomitant features. When cervical spondylosis causes cord compression, the principal differentiation is from demyelinating disease. Depression may occur secondary to any painful disorder, but it may itself be a contributory cause of chronic spinal pain.

Investigation

Radiology of the neck and chest, together with estimation of haemoglobin, white cell count, ESR and bone biochemistry, are mandatory investigations for persistent spinal pain. Most people develop narrowing and intervertebral osteophytes of the lower-most cervical intervertebral joints and such changes may have no relevance to symptoms.

Investigations may be entirely normal in neck strain and cervical disc prolapse. In cervical spondylosis the radiological evidence of OA associated with ageing tends to be more severe and widespread although some patients with chronic pain have normal radiographs. In these cases the term cervical spondylosis is used to describe a syndrome rather than a pathological entity. The presence of cervical ribs is usually irrelevant to neck and arm symptoms.

A high ESR may denote polymyalgia rheumatica, malignant disease or infection. An early radiographic feature of malignancy is disappearance of a vertebral pedicle (*Figure 6.1*). Destruction of a vertebral body and disc space suggest an infectious process and soft tissue shadowing anterior to the vertebrae an associated

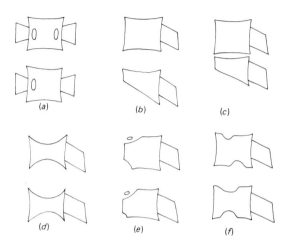

Figure 6.1   Appearance of spinal radiographs. (a) Antero-posterior view showing loss of a pedicle in malignant disease; (b) collapse of vertebral body with preservation of disc space due to malignancy or metabolic bone disease; (c) vertebral collapse with loss of adjacent disc, a picture which is highly suggestive of spinal infection; (d) biconcave (codfish) vertebrae in metabolic bone disease; (e) wedging of vertebrae due to Scheuermann's disease; (f) Schmorl's nodes

abscess. Collapse or destruction of only the vertebra is indicative of neoplastic or metabolic bone disease. Sclerosis of a vertebra may represent a secondary deposit from prostate, breast, lymphoma, thyroid or other viscera. A sclerotic vertebra which is also enlarged is likely to be involved by Paget's disease. A high serum alkaline phosphatase may support a diagnosis of either Paget's disease or malignancy of bone. Hypercalcaemia may be a feature of widespread skeletal metastases or multiple myeloma.

Where serious underlying disease is suspected and radiographs are normal, a technetium bone scan may demonstrate one or more skeletal lesions. Needle biopsy may be necessary to secure a diagnosis of infection or malignancy. Evidence of cervical cord compression may be confirmed by myelography. Nerve conduction studies may be necessary to distinguish carpal tunnel syndrome from cervical nerve root entrapment.

Aetiology

Neck strain

This is invariably caused by tearing of muscle or ligamentous attachments with secondary inflammation as healing proceeds.

Cervical disc prolapse

The cause is usually not apparent. Coughing, straining or unaccustomed physical activity may be significant factors.

Cervical spondylosis

There may be a history of past trauma or a predisposition to generalized osteoarthritis as manifest by clinical evidence of peripheral arthritis. It occurs from middle age onwards.

Pathology

Cervical disc protrusion

This tends to occur in young and middle aged subjects in whom the nucleus pulposus retains its gelatinous texture. Protrusion occurs through the thin posterior longitudinal ligament most often in a postero-lateral direction. Impingement of the disc on an emerging nerve root excites an inflammatory response around the nerve (*Figure 6.2*).

Cervical spondylosis

The ageing changes of the intervertebral discs result in a gradual loss of their height and a decreased ability to absorb pressure. This predisposes to the development of osteoarthritis which occurs at intervertebral and facetal joints. The histological features are the same as those of osteoarthritis at other sites (*see* Chapter 4). Large posterior osteophytes may encroach on the spinal canal.

Treatment

The aim of treatment is symptomatic. Pain may be alleviated or modified by simple analgesics and anti-inflammatory drugs. Adequate sleep is important because tiredness can accentuate depression and pain. One pillow is better than several, a soft collar for nocturnal use may help, and occasionally hypnotics are warranted. Rest of the neck is important and may be achieved with a firm collar.

Physical treatments such as traction, heat, manipulation and exercises may provide transient symptomatic relief. These benefits may be no more than a placebo response, but they are nevertheless worthwhile.

Surgery is indicated only where there is cord compression. Laminectomy and discectomy may prevent progression but some neurological deficit usually persists.

Course

Neck strain symptoms usually resolve within two weeks although whiplash injuries may cause symptoms which persist for months.

Symptoms from cervical disc protrusions usually resolve over a period of 2–4 months.

Cervical spondylosis is associated with persistent or intermittent discomfort. Many patients adapt to their symptoms but others, especially those beset with social or psychological difficulties, may become totally preoccupied by their pain.

Dorsal pain

Pain in the dorsal spine is less fequent than in the neck and lumbar regions. Strain, disc protrusions and osteoarthritis may occur and the symptoms, signs and treatment are similar to those described for the neck. Root involvement causes pain which radiates around the chest wall.

In older children and adolescents, dorsal pain may be caused by Scheuermann's disease in which pain may be associated with progressive kyphosis of the dorsal spine. Radiographs show characteristic anterior wedging of the vertebral bodies due to separation of the ring epiphyses by intervertebral discs. More centrally placed indentations caused by discs are referred to as Schmorl's nodes. The latter are radiological features which occur in both dorsal and lumbar regions, usually in the absence of symptoms (*Figure 6.1*).

In older patients the differential diagnosis of dorsal back pain also includes metabolic bone disease and diffuse idiopathic skeletal hyperostosis (*see* p. 64).

Lumbar pain

Low back pain has several well recognized causes but the majority of patients have symptoms which cannot be easily explained in mechanical or pathological terms. These are categorized as non-specific low back pain.

Symptoms

Non-specific back pain

Pain and stiffness may develop insidiously or suddenly. There may be a history of rigorous physical activity or sustained abnormal posture such as may be encountered in long car journeys, gardening or decorating. Symptoms often occur a day after the precipitating event. There may be some referral of pain into the buttock, but more distant referral, impulse pain and neurological symptoms are absent. Stiffness may be more severe in the morning.

Lumbar disc protrusion

The onset may resemble that of non-specific back pain and there may be a long history of intermittent mild backache. A history of subsequent pain, paraesthesiae or numbness in a leg is highly suggestive of lumbar disc protusion. Referred discomfort may be sciatic in distribution or, less commonly, follow the femoral nerve supply. Pain on straining or coughing (impulse pain) is usual. Occasionally patients may complain of foot drop.

Lumbar spondylosis

Osteoarthritis of the spine is a cause of chronic or intermittent low back pain, usually with little or no root symptoms. The history may be indistinguishable from that of non-specific low back pain.

Leg pain induced by walking and relieved by rest in the presence of a good peripheral circulation suggests intermittent claudication of the cauda equina. This is a feature of spinal stenosis, a problem which is most often a complication of lumbar spondylosis.

Spondylolysis and spondylolisthesis

Pain may be abrupt or slow in onset. Root symptoms may occur even in the absence of disc degeneration. Symptoms of intermittent claudication of the cauda equina may also be apparent.

Signs

A scoliosis is common but may have more than one cause. It may be:

1. congenital;
2. due to muscle spasm;
3. an attempt to relieve a compressed nerve root; or
4. compensation for pelvic tilting due to a short leg.

Paravertebral muscle spasm is usual in patients with back pain of any cause. This causes a rigid spine with loss of the normal lordosis and a restricted range of forward flexion. Tenderness of the vertebrae, paravertebral structures, sacroiliac and other pelvic areas are common but non-specific features of back pain.

Restriction of straight leg raising may simply reflect muscle spasm, but pronounced limitation, associated worsening of neurological symptoms or pain on lifting the contralateral leg are indicative of sciatic nerve root compression. A positive femoral nerve stretch test suggests femoral nerve root impingement.

Specific nerve root lesions may be manifest by wasting of quadricep or diminished knee reflex (L3, 4), weakness of ankle dorsiflexion (L4), weakness of the extensor hallucis, other toe extensors or foot eversion (L5), diminished or absent ankle reflex (S1) and sensory impairment in the L4 or L5 root distributions.

Differential diagnosis

Non-specific back pain, disc prolapse, spondylosis and spondylolysis have to be distinguished from the infectious malignant diseases discussed for neck pain.

Rheumatoid arthritis does not materially affect the lower spine but ankylosing spondylitis and sacroiliitis characteristically present with low pack pain. Nocturnal pain and pronounced morning stiffness are suggestive of sacroiliitis or spondylitis but are by no means diagnostic.

Metabolic bone diseases and diffuse idiopathic skeletal hyperostosis are additional causes of low back pain which are discussed below.

Pain in the buttock may be associated with any of the spinal disorders but may also be caused by hip disease, sacroiliitis, ischial or trochanteric bursitis. The distinction is not always easy and depends on eliciting additional signs of spinal, sacroiliac or hip disease.

Neurological symptoms and signs due to spinal pathology sometimes arise in the absence of back pain or persist when such symptoms have resolved. Distinction from primary neurological disorders such as motor neurone disease may occasionally require further investigation.

Symptoms of intermittent claudication of the cauda equina may be identical to the pain of peripheral vascular disease. Distinction is especially difficult when peripheral pulses are absent and investigation may then involve arteriography. In addition to lumbar spondylosis and spondylolisthesis, Paget's disease and intraspinal tumours may cause cauda equina claudication.

Coccydinia is a painful disorder confined to the coccyx and is most often seen after child delivery. It tends to resolve spontaneously after many months.

Intra-abdominal pathology such as pancreatic disease and pelvic inflammation are rare non-spinal causes of low back pain.

Investigations

Persistent lumbar pain must be investigated by the same routine haematological and biochemical tests described for the neck.

Radiographs of the spine are essential for the exclusion of infections and malignant disease, the features of which are described in the section on the cervical spine (*see Figure 6.1*). Vertebral collapse in the lumbar region may also be due to osteoporosis. Clinical or laboratory evidence of serious disease in the presence of normal radiographs can be further investigated by bone scan and needle biopsy.

A radiograph of the pelvis is essential because low back pain may derive from the sacroiliac joints or other areas of the pelvis. It may also provide further evidence of metabolic bone disease.

In lumbar disc prolapse the radiographs are often normal. Confirmation of root compression may be obtained by a radiculogram, venogram or CT scan. These investigations are usually warranted when symptoms are persistent and surgery is contemplated. Radiculography or CT scan may also be used to confirm spinal stenosis.

Narrowing of the lumbosacral joint with or without osteophytes is common and not always related to symptoms.

Congenital anomalies of the lumbosacral region occur in 5% of the population. The fifth lumbar vertebra (L5) may articulate with one or both iliac bones (sacralization). Spondylolysis and spina bifida occulta may occur alone or with sacralization of L5. These findings are not usually painful but both unilateral sacralization of L5 and spondylolysis may be associated with back pain. The latter represents a defect in the pars interarticularis of L4 or 5 and is best visualized on oblique views of the spine.

Forward slipping of a lower lumbar vertebra is termed spondylolisthesis and this may follow a spondylolysis or osteoarthritis of the intervertebral and facetal joints.

Aetiology

Non-specific back pain

This occurs in young and middle aged subjects. A history of unaccustomed physical activity, sustained periods of abnormal posture or acute strains can usually be elicited.

Lumbar disc protrusion

The same age range and activities described for non-specific back pain are relevant. In addition, the lifting or pulling of heavy loads can often be incriminated.

Lumbar spondylosis

This condition occurs in middle to old age. Acute lumbar disc protrusions are uncommon in the elderly. Men are more susceptible, particularly those who have engaged in heavy work. There may be a previous history of acute lumbar disc protrusion.

Any disorder which causes a chronic lumbar scoliosis will alter the mechanical forces and predispose to the development of spondylosis. Congenital kyphoscoliosis, and disparities of leg length, are two examples of this.

Lumbar spondylolysis and spondylolisthesis

It is not certain what proportion of pars interarticularis defects are present at birth. An association with other spinal malformations suggests that a defect or at least a structural weakness may be congenital. An unknown number of pars defects are traumatic and represent stress fractures. These are most common amongst young people engaged in athletic pursuits.

The presence of bilateral spondylolysis removes the restraining influence of the inferior facetal joints and forward subluxation or spondylolisthesis may result (*see Figure 6.2*). Spondylolisthesis may also occur in lumbar spondylosis because of realignment of articulating surfaces due to bone remodelling of the facets and loss of intervertebral joint space.

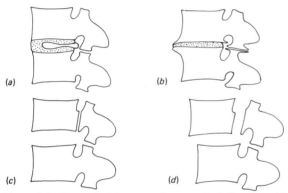

Figure 6.2   Anatomical features of some spinal disorders. (a) Disc prolapse; (b) spondylosis (osteoarthritis of the spine); (c) pars interarticularis defect (spondylolysis); (d) forward subluxation of a vertebra (spondylolisthesis)

Pathology

Non-specific low back pain

In the absence of clinical, radiological or laboratory evidence of specific pathology it is presumed that pain derives from ligaments or muscles attached to the vertebrae or from the facetal joints. Tears, haematoma and inflammation probably constitute the spectrum of pathology although in any individual case these are speculative changes.

Lumbar disc protrusion and lumbar spondylosis

These are associated with the same pathology described for the respective cervical disorders (*see Figure 6.2*).

Treatment

Non-specific back pain

Rest and analgesics are all that are required for the majority. Recurrent or persistent symptoms may benefit from one or other of the many physical treatments outlined in the section on neck pain, including spinal manipulation. None of these alters the natural history of back ache but the placebo effect of treatment administered by a therapist is often worthwhile. A lumbar corset may be helpful for those with chronic symptoms, and areas of well-defined tenderness may be responsive to injections of local anaesthetic and corticosteroid.

Reassurance and adequate sleep are important but it sometimes becomes clear that patients with chronic or intermittent pain are depressed or have some other psychiatric illness. It is not always possible to determine whether the pain preceded evidence of mental distress. A sympathetic hearing and judicious use of antidepressants or hypnotics may be helpful but perseverance is often demanded of both patient and physician.

Education on caring for the back may prevent or limit recurrence. This may involve attention to posture at rest or work, an awareness of risk factors, a firm bed and improved physical fitness.

Lumbar disc protrusion

Rest in bed is the best treatment. For those who wish to remain active, provision of a corset may be helpful. Analgesics, hypnotics, reassurance and education have the same value as for non-specific back pain.

Pain which remains disabling or is not improving after at least one week of complete bed rest and several weeks of restricted activity may warrant additional treatment. Rapid restoration of fitness is crucial to those earning a living for their family. Hospital admission may allow supervised rest. One or more epidural injections of corticosteroid diluted in normal saline may accelerate improvement.

If disability persists despite these measures, radiographic confirmation of the site of the lesion should precede surgical referral. Removal of the offending nucleus pulposus may be achieved at laminectomy or by discectomy. Chemonucleolysis by the injection of chymopapain into the disc is an alternative procedure which may become more widely used than at present.

Lumbar spondylosis

Symptoms are not usually progressive nor necessarily chronic. The symptomatic measures used to treat non-specific back pain can be applied with somewhat less expectation of sustained improvement. Where scoliosis is secondary to leg shortening a shoe raise may alleviate some of the symptoms. Surgery has a small role. Osteoarthritis confined to one level may benefit from vertebral fusion. Spinal stenosis, however, is a firm indication for operative decompression of the spinal canal.

Spondylolysis and spondylolisthesis

Rest and provision of a corset may improve pain especially when a pars defect represents a fracture of recent onset. Unremitting pain associated with a pars defect may improve with surgical stabilization. Similar surgery for spondylolisthesis is often disappointing because of secondary OA or damage to neighbouring structures. Where spondylolisthesis is clearly due to spondylosis in the absence of a pars interarticularis defect there is no place for surgery. If there are associated symptoms of intermittent claudication of the cauda equina, surgical decompression may be required.

Course

Non-specific back pain improves within four weeks in more than 90% of patients. A chronic or relapsing course is confined to a minority.

Acute lumbar disc protrusion pain also remits with conservative measures in about 90% within 2–3 months. Some patients experience recurrent disc lesions at the same or adjacent sites. Persistent pain in patients with suggestive histories of disc protrusion, especially in those who have undergone myelography with insoluble contrast material or laminectomy, may have arachnoiditis. This is caused by scarring and tethering of nerve root sheaths and has no certain remedy.

Spondylolysis and spondylolisthesis may both be asymptomatic findings and if surgery is contemplated for pain, alternative causes need to be first excluded.

Diffuse idiopathic skeletal hyperostosis (DISH, Vertebral Ankylosing Hyperostosis, Forestier's Disease)

This is essentially a radiographic entity and is often asymptomatic. It is characterized by large vertebral osteophytes which, unlike the horizontal outgrowths of spondylosis, extend vertically to bridge the intervertebral spaces, superficially resembling ankylosing spondylitis. The osteophytes are much thicker than those of lumbar spondylosis and the syndesmophytes of ankylosing spondylitis. The disc spaces are often of normal height, another feature distinguishing it from spondylosis (*Figure 6.3*). The

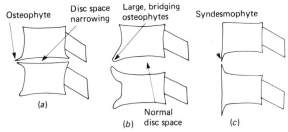

Figure 6.3 Appearance of lateral radiographs of the spine. (a) Osteoarthritis (spondylosis); (b) diffuse idiopathic skeletal hyperostosis; (c) ankylosing spondylitis

sacroiliac joints and laboratory indices of inflammation are normal and there is no association with any tissue antigen. The findings are most obvious in the dorsal region but both the cervical and lumbar spines may be involved. At other skeletal sites there may be ragged new bone formation where muscles or fascia are attached.

The condition is much more common in the elderly and there is an association with diabetes mellitus and acromegaly. If present, symptoms are confined to mild spinal stiffness and pain but examination may reveal dorsal kyphosis and restricted spinal movement. No specific treatment is indicated.

Further reading

B.A.P.M. (1966). Pain in the neck and arm – a multicentre trial of the effects of physiotherapy. *Br. Med. J.*, **1**, 253

DEYO, R. (1983). Conservative therapy for low back pain – distinguishing useful from useless therapy. *J. Am. Med. Ass.*, **250**, 1057

FRYMOYER, J. *et al.* (1983). Risk factors in low back pain – an epidemiological survey. *J. Bone Jt. Surg.*, **65A**, 213

LAWRENCE, J. (1969). Disc degeneration. Its frequency and relationship to symptoms. *Ann. Rheum. Dis.*, **28**, 121

LIPSON, S. *et al.* (1981). Experimental intervertebral disc degeneration – morphologic and proteoglycan changes over time. *Arthritis Rheum.*, **24**, 12

7
Metabolic bone disease

Pain in the spine or at other skeletal sites may be due to osteoporotic vertebral collapse, osteomalacia, hyperparathyroidism or Paget's disease.

Osteoporosis

This disorder is one of diminished bone mass.

Symptoms

There may be radiological evidence of osteoporosis and even slow collapse of vertebrae without any history of discomfort. However, sudden vertebral collapse invariably causes acute pain at the site of abnormality. The risk of fractures is increased and the femoral neck and wrist are vulnerable sites.

Signs

In many elderly subjects with progressive vertebral wedging, there may be loss of height, dorsal kyphosis but little or no tenderness. Acute crush fractures, on the other hand, are associated with pronounced tenderness, muscle spasm and restriction of lumbar or dorsal movement. Cord or nerve root signs occur rarely.

Differential diagnosis

The other causes of vertebral collapse discussed in Chapter 6 need to be considered. Myelomatosis may cause diffuse loss of bone density. Pathological fractures caused by metastatic malignancy may require exclusion. Osteomalacia causes similar loss of radiological osteopenia and may be difficult to distinguish if bone biochemistry is normal and if both radiographs and bone scans fail to reveal Looser zones.

Investigation

Radiographs show reduced density of both trabecular and medullary bone. These changes may be localized to areas of disuse. Views of the spine may show wedging or biconcave collapse of lumbar or dorsal vertebrae (codfish spine) (see Figure 6.1(d)).

Bone scans are normal unless there have been recent fractures or vertebral collapse. Quantification of osteoporosis by neutron activation analysis of total body bone mass and photon absorption of specific sites have limited research applications. CT scanning techniques may give the most accurate assessment of bone mineral content. Haematological and biochemical investigations are normal.

Aetiology

Loss of bone mass occurs with ageing and is more pronounced in elderly females than males because males have larger and denser skeletons. In females, the condition accelerates after menopause because of the lost anabolic effect of oestrogens.

Occasionally the disorder affects young people without an obvious explanation. Testosterone deficiency, thyrotoxicosis, rheumatoid arthritis, corticosteroid treatment, disuse and immobilization are all acknowledged causes. In senile and some other patterns of osteoporosis there is evidence of reduced calcium absorption but it is uncertain whether this is of aetiological importance.

Pathology

Unlike osteomalacia, mineralization is normal. Attempts to interpret biopsy material dynamically suggest that bone resorption and bone formation may be altered to varying extents depending on aetiology.

Treatment

Spinal pain due to vertebral collapse can be effectively managed by analgesics and bed rest. A corset may help those with persistent lumbar discomfort. There is no treatment which can restore senile or postmenopausal osteoporosis to a healthier state. Disuse, corticosteroid-induced and thyrotoxic osteoporosis may improve after elimination of the cause. Oestrogen replacement in postmenopausal patients can lessen the rate of further progression but carries a risk of vaginal bleeding, vascular thrombosis, hypertension and possibly uterine carcinoma. There is no good evidence that supplements of calcium, vitamin D or sodium fluoride are beneficial.

Course

Acute spinal pain treated by rest improves within 1–2 weeks. The elderly population with progressive osteoporosis is, in general, not disabled by persistent pain or spinal deformity.

Osteomalacia

This is a disorder in which there is a failure to mineralize normal bone mass.

Symptoms

Although pathological fractures and vertebral collapse occasionally give rise to severe pain in osteomalacia, it is more usual for patients to present with diffuse skeletal discomfort. Muscle weakness may be an important component and impaired walking may be caused by a combination of bone pain and weakness.

Signs

In rickets, the childhood equivalent of osteomalacia, bone deformity of legs, arms, skull and rib cage are common but these are not features of the adult disease. Bone tenderness of spine and extremities may be apparent but is mild. Weakness of proximal muscles is an important sign. The characteristic waddling gait is mainly caused by weakness of hip muscles although pelvic pain may be contributory. When hypocalcaemia is apparent, tetany, a positive Chvostek's or Trousseau's sign may be demonstrable.

Differential diagnosis

The principal difficulty is in distinguishing the generalized loss of bone density from that of osteoporosis. When myopathic features are pronounced, other causes of proximal myopathy such as hypothyroidism, myositis and diabetes mellitus may require exclusion.

Investigation

Skeletal radiology should be confined to sites of pain or to areas where Looser zones are likely to be found. These are segments of demineralized bone and although sometimes referred to as Milkman fractures, they are not true fractures. They are seen in the pelvis, the long bones of arms and legs, especially around the femoral neck, the axillary borders of the scapulae and the ribs (*Figure 7.1*).

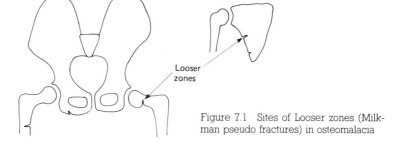

Looser zones

Figure 7.1   Sites of Looser zones (Milkman pseudo fractures) in osteomalacia

Bone scans may reveal the sites of Looser zones not initially apparent on radiographs. The avidity of the skeleton for technetium or other isotopes which accumulate in bone may be calculated from clearance rates and these may be of value in diagnosis.

The serum alkaline phosphatase is elevated in more than 90% of patients. Serum calcium may be low or at the lower range of normal. Serum phosphate may be reduced, occasionally in the presence of normal calcium values. Such patients may have hypophosphataemic osteomalacia which is caused by renal phosphate wasting. Urine calcium levels are usually reduced and, if secondary hyperparathyroidism is present, excretion of hydroxyproline may be increased.

Measurements of vitamin D metabolites in the circulation may provide confirmatory evidence of vitamin D deficiency. Bone biopsy is a useful means of confirming the diagnosis but interpretation may be difficult.

Aetiology

An appreciation of vitamin D metabolism is useful for an understanding of osteomalacia (*Figure 7.2*). One source of vitamin D_3 is the action of ultraviolet light on 7-dehydrocholesterol in the skin. Calcium homeostasis is achieved partly by the action of

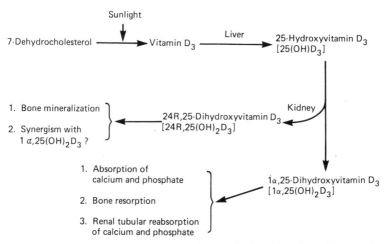

Figure 7.2 The metabolism of vitamin D showing the hepatic and renal stages of hydroxylation

$1\alpha,25$-dihydroxyvitamin D_3, the synthesis of which is increased by the kidney during hypocalcaemia. This effect is mediated by the action of parathyroid hormone (PTH). Hypercalcaemia and hyperphosphataemia have a suppressant effect on the renal hydroxylation of vitamin D_3. Synthesis of $1\alpha,25$-dihydroxyvitamin D_3 declines with age and is one explanation for the decreased gut absorption of calcium which accompanies ageing. The metabolite

24R, 25-dihydroxyvitamin D_3 is also produced by the kidney and its synthesis is promoted by 1α,25-dihydroxyvitamin D_3 and suppressed by PTH. The interaction of vitamin D metabolites and their precise roles remain controversial.

The disease is most often due to dietary deficiency or malabsorption of vitamin D. It is more common in areas of poverty and malnutrition. In Britain, rickets was frequent in urban areas before the development of the welfare state. Both rickets and osteomalacia are now more or less confined to Asian immigrants. The reasons for this racial localization are probably multifactorial and include lack of exposure to ultraviolet light, dietary deficiency of vitamin D and binding of calcium to phytate contained in chapati flour.

Malabsorption of vitamin D may occur in diseases of the small bowel, liver, pancreas or in blind loop syndrome following partial gastrectomy. Patients in renal failure may develop osteomalacia as part of the picture of renal osteodystrophy. Inadequate hydroxylation to 1α,25-dihydroxyvitamin D_3 accounts for some but not all cases.

Hypophosphataemia is most often due to phosphate-losing nephropathy. Several types of this disorder have been documented and they are often described as cases of vitamin D-resistant rickets.

Renal dialysis may cause osteomalacia by absorption of aluminium from the dialysate. This becomes preferentially substituted for calcium in bone.

Osteomalacia may be caused by long-term phenytoin treatment. This drug lowers 25-hydroxyvitamin D_3 levels by inducing increased hepatic catabolism. However, 1α,25-dihydroxyvitamin D_3 levels are not affected so the relevance of this observation is uncertain.

Pathology

The main feature is a widening of the unossified osteoid seam. Labelling of bone with fluorescent tetracycline two weeks before a biopsy allows assessment of the rate of mineralization which is reduced in osteomalacia.

Treatment

Correction of dietary deficiency with supplements of vitamin D will be adequate where intake or absorption is abnormal. In malabsorption vitamin D is best given parenterally. Use of the 1α,25-dihydroxyvitamin D_3 preparation is more likely to be effective in renal failure.

Course

Symptomatic, biochemical and radiological improvement are usually apparent within a few weeks of vitamin D treatment, except in hypophosphataemia and some cases of renal osteodystrophy.

Primary hyperparathyroidism

This may cause rheumatic symptoms by several mechanisms.

Symptoms

The classical symptoms of polydipsia, polyuria, renal colic and bone pain are now uncommon presenting symptoms. It is more likely for the diagnosis to be suspected on the basis of incidentally detected hypercalcaemia in an asymptomatic patient.

The earliest symptoms of hyperparathyroidism are vague bone, joint and muscle pain, weakness and malaise. Acute joint pain and swelling due to pseudogout may occur. Sustained hypercalcaemia may cause anorexia, nausea and constipation. Pronounced hypercalcaemia may result in pancreatitis, mental confusion or coma.

Signs

There may be demonstrable muscle weakness without wasting or tenderness. Acute pseudogout with warmth, swelling and effusion may affect knee, wrist or other joints. Calcification of the conjunctiva or cornea may be apparent on inspection but slit lamp examination is required to exclude this finding. There is an association with hypertension.

Differential diagnosis

In most patients the disease has to be distinguished from other causes of hypercalcaemia, the most common cause of which is malignant disease with skeletal involvement. Other possibilities include sarcoidosis, vitamin D intoxication, diuretic therapy and tumours secreting polypeptides resembling PTH, prostaglandins, cyclic AMP or other osteoclast-activating substances. Symptomatic hyperparathyroidism may resemble early inflammatory joint disease, osteoarthritis, myositis or the musculoskeletal symptoms of hypothyroidism.

Investigation

The finding of a raised serum calcium and low phosphate is very suggestive of hyperparathyroidism. Phosphate levels are reduced in about 50% and serum alkaline phosphatase may be raised.

The steroid suppression test involves giving hydrocortisone 40 mg three times daily for ten days and will suppress hypercalcaemia in most disorders other than hyperparathyroidism.

Urine calcium tends to be low and phosphate high for their respective serum levels. Estimation of the tubular phosphate reabsorption to GFR ratio is usually low.

Measurement of PTH will reveal levels which are undisputedly high or in the high normal range. Most other causes of hypercalcaemia reduce PTH.

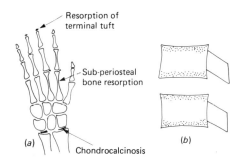

Figure 7.3 Characteristic radiographic appearance of (a) the hand in hyperparathyroidism; and (b) the spine in renal osteodystrophy. The sclerotic margins produce the characteristic 'rugger jersey spine'

Radiographs of the hands may reveal sub-periosteal or terminal tuft resorption (*Figure 7.3(a)*). Views of peripheral joints may demonstrate chondrocalcinosis, notably of the knees and wrists. In late disease, cysts may arise in long bones (brown tumours). When warranted by the history, plain abdominal or IVU radiographs may demonstrate renal calculi or nephrocalcinosis.

Persistent hypercalcaemia may lead to impairment of GFR and an increased serum creatinine. Hyperuricaemia is often present, presumably due to renal tubular impairment.

Parathyroid adenoma may be demonstrated by subtraction isotope techniques using thallium and technetium.

Aetiology

The majority of patients with primary hyperparathyroidism have a single adenoma. Less than 10% have hyperplasia or parathyroid carcinoma. The excess PTH stimulates osteoclasts to resorb bone, accentuates intestinal absorption of calcium and increases calcium tubular reabsorption. It has an opposite effect on phosphate handling.

Pathology

In advanced disease, cystic changes may occur in bone. These may be haemorrhagic and this accounts for the old pathological term, brown tumours. Bone is histologically normal apart from increased numbers of osteoclasts.

Treatment

The increasing recognition of asymptomatic and mild cases has led to a more circumspect therapeutic approach. If such cases have good renal function they are best observed. Patients who have severe symptoms, renal calculi or impaired GFR warrant neck exploration and removal of abnormal parathyroid tissue.

Course

Symptoms directly related to hypercalcaemia remit within days of surgical treatment. Muscle weakness and bone pain improve over weeks but joint symptoms may persist. Radiological evidence of bone resorption is halted but chondrocalcinosis continues to progress.

Renal osteodystrophy

This is a combination of osteomalacia and secondary hyperparathyroidism occurring in renal failure. One or other of these disorders may dominate the clinical picture.

The symptoms, signs and pathology constitute a variable spectrum which covers the features described for osteomalacia and hyperparathyroidism.

Differential diagnosis

The differential diagnosis includes avascular necrosis if patients are receiving corticosteroids for their renal disease.

Investigation

Investigation may reveal high or low serum calcium, elevated serum phosphate, high alkaline phosphatase and raised PTH. Circulating $1\alpha,25$-dihydroxyvitamin D_3 and $24R,25$-dihydroxyvitamin D_3 are reduced.

The radiological changes of both osteomalacia and hyperparathyroidism may be present. In addition, osteosclerosis may occur. This feature is poorly understood and most frequently affects the margins of the vertebral bodies, giving rise to the so-called 'rugger jersey spine' (*Figure 7.3(b)*).

Aetiology

The aetiology of renal osteodystrophy is due to a failure of the kidney to hydroxylate vitamin D_3. The hyperparathyroidism is a secondary response to the resultant hypocalcaemia.

Treatment

Most patients respond to supplements of $1\alpha,25$-dihydroxyvitamin D_3 but a few do not. The reason for this is not clear. Patients with marked hyperparathyroidism usually have gross parathyroid hyperplasia but some develop an autonomous adenoma (tertiary hyperparathyroidism). In both cases parathyroidectomy is the best therapeutic approach.

Paget's disease

This is a disease of unknown aetiology which causes enlargement, softening and deformity of bone.

Symptoms

The majority of patients with Paget's disease are asymptomatic. Bone pain is the principal complaint. Pain may also arise from fractures of involved sites, osteoarthritis of adjacent joints and vertebral collapse. Spinal involvement may cause root symptoms or intermittent claudication of the cauda equina. Skull involvement may rarely be associated with deafness and other cranial nerve symptoms.

Signs

Involved sites may be warm due to increased vascularity of bone and overlying skin. Deformities due to increase of bone size and alterations of alignment are common. Bowing of the tibiae and femurs is characteristic (*Figure 7.4(a)*).

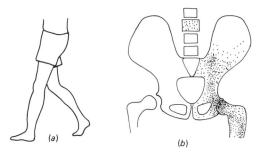

Figure 7.4   Paget's disease (a) involving the left tibia to cause a typical bowing appearance, and (b) affecting the pelvis, left femur and third lumbar vertebra. Note the patchy sclerotic appearance, enlargement of involved bone and the secondary osteoarthritis of the hip joint

Skull disease is manifest by enlargement of the head with frontal bossing. Cranial nerve involvement is uncommon and platybasia may be associated with signs of medullary cord compression. Vertebral involvement may cause nerve root signs and local tenderness. Associated OA of hip or knee may be confirmed by restricted movement. Determining whether pain is due mainly to the joint disease or underlying Paget's involvement may be difficult. In severe widespread disease there may be evidence of high output congestive heart failure. Angioid streaking of the retina is occasionally observed.

Rapid worsening of pain, especially when associated with swelling, may denote the development of osteosarcoma.

Differential diagnosis

The important distinction is from sclerotic malignant deposits, the most common source of which is the prostate in men and the breast in women. Enlargement of bone is consistent with Paget's disease but not malignancy.

Fibrous dysplasia is a rare disorder of bone which has some radiological resemblance to Paget's disease.

Investigation

The diagnosis is often established incidentally on the basis of routine radiology. Initially there may be coarsening of trabeculation. Areas of dense sclerosis may develop alongside relatively lytic areas (*Figure 7.4(b)*). Enlargement of bone and deformity such as wedging of vertebrae or bowing of long bones may be apparent radiologically. The skull may show thickening of the vault and a typical mottled appearance. Bone scans may demonstrate involvement which is equivocal on radiographs. Scanning may also be a guide to disease activity during treatment.

Routine haematology, serum and urine calcium and phosphate are all normal. Hypercalcaemia rarely develops after immobilization. Serum alkaline phosphatase increases when there is sufficient bone disease and the level reflects both the activity and the extent of skeleton affected. Urine hydroxyproline excretion is increased and correlates with the level of serum alkaline phosphatase. Serum acid phosphatase is usually normal, a feature which may help to distinguish the disease from prostatic carcinoma.

Bone biopsy is hardly ever warranted except where sarcomatous change is suspected.

Aetiology

Males are more susceptible than females and the majority of patients present after the age of 60.

There is geographical variation in prevalence, the disease being more common in some parts of Britain such as Lancashire and rare in Japan and China. There is no certain familial association nor is there a link with any HLA antigen. The cause is unknown but the finding of inclusion bodies in osteoclasts has raised the possiblity of a viral aetiology. Measles virus has been implicated but the evidence is controversial.

Pathology

The initial changes result from osteoclast activity. The resorption of bone accounts for the increased excretion of hydroxyproline. Osteoblastic activity increases to match that of the osteoclasts and this elevates the serum alkaline phosphatase. The bone becomes soft and the resorption area is expanded. The osteoclasts contain more nuclei than normal and inclusions of hydroxyapatite crystals may be defined. The osteoblasts are increased in size. Bone turnover increases many times and the bone becomes highly vascular due to increased numbers of arterioles.

Treatment

Mild pain can be successfully contained by simple analgesics and non-steroidal anti-inflammatory drugs. A corset may help lumbar pain. Severe pain, deformity or complications warrant treatment with calcitonin or diphosphonate.

Calcitonin inhibits bone resorption and is given parenterally three times weekly for 8–12 months. Nausea and other gastrointestinal disturbances are common.

Diphosphonates inhibit both bone resorption and mineralization. Of these only disodium etidronate is generally available and is given as a single oral dose daily for six months. Gastrointestinal side effects are common and prolonged treatment will cause osteomalacia and an increased rate of fractures. Both calcitonin and diphosphonates may relieve bone pain within days or weeks. An effect on serum alkaline phosphatase and bone scan activity may be apparent within the first week. There may be some advantage in using both drugs in combination.

Mithramycin is a cytotoxic agent which can rapidly abolish pain due to Paget's disease. Biochemical evidence of disease activity is also reduced. It is administered by intravenous infusion but repeated applications are hazardous because of adverse effects on liver, kidney and marrow function.

If severe osteoarthritis develops, joint replacement is not precluded although technically the arthroplasty may be more difficult and the outcome less certain because of the soft bone.

Course

Intermittent courses of anti-Paget's treatment can, to a large extent, modify the symptoms. In widespread or severe disease an awareness of the risk of sarcoma must be maintained.

Further reading

DETHERIDGE, F. *et al.* (1982). European distribution of Paget's disease of bone. *Br. Med. J.,* **285,** 1005

EDITORIAL (1985). Risk factors in postmenopausal osteoporosis. *Lancet,* **1,** 1370

HOSKING, D. *et al.* (1983). Screening for subclinical osteomalacia in the elderly: normal ranges or pragmatism. *Lancet,* **2,** 1290

KRANE, S. (1982). Etidronate disodium in the treatment of Paget's disease of bone. *Ann. Med.,* **96,** 619

SHARMAN, V. *et al.* (1982). Long term experience of alfacalcidol in renal osteodystrophy. *Q. J. Med.,* **51,** 271

WHYTE, M. *et al.* (1982). Postmenopausal osteoporosis – a heterogeneous disorder as assessed by histomorphometric analysis of iliac crest bone from untreated patients. *Am. J. Med.,* **72,** 193

8
Spondylarthritis

The diseases described in this chapter (ankylosing spondylitis, psoriatic arthropathy, reactive arthritis and enteropathic arthritis) may be aassociated with a predominantly large joint arthritis, sacroiliitis and spondylitis. The heading spondylarthritis can therefore be legitimately applied to this group of conditions but with some qualification. The majority of patients with psoriatic and enteropathic arthritis have a type of disorder which is not associated with sacroiliitis. In general, it is only those who possess HLA B27 who are susceptible to this manifestation.

The term 'seronegative arthritis' is often used to describe these and other non-rheumatoid inflammatory joint disorders. It is an unsatisfactory expression because (a) not all cases of RA are seropositive, i.e. have a positive test for IgM RF, and (b) many disorders are seronegative but have no common aetiological or clinical features. In order to avoid ambiguity and to discourage students using the term as though it were a precise diagnosis, it is not used in this book.

Ankylosing spondylitis

This is an arthritis which predominantly affects the spine and sacroiliac joints. Classically, it is a disease of young men.

Symptoms

Symptoms begin insidiously, usually with low back pain and stiffness. Pain may be referred into a buttock but sciatica is not usually a feature. Both pain and stiffness are characteristically worse in the morning or after inactivity. Nocturnal pain may disturb sleep. These features are suggestive but not diagnostic of ankylosing spondylitis. Pain occasionally begins in the neck, dorsal spine, chest or a peripheral joint. Asymmetrical pain and swelling of ankles or knees should always suggest spondylarthritis. Peripheral arthritis occurs in 30% of patients with spondylitis. Heel pain due to plantar fasciitis is seen in 10%.

Soreness and redness of an eye may indicate the presence of iritis. A history of recurrent abdominal pain or diarrhoea suggests associated inflammatory bowel disease. Psoriasis, previous enteritis or a history of urethritis may imply that spondylitis is a manifestation of psoriatic or reactive arthritis.

Signs

In early disease, when inflammation is localized to the sacroiliac joints, there may be few signs. Restriction of lumbosacral movement may be slight. In later disease, rigidity may become more pronounced so that flexion takes place at the hips (*Figure 8.1*). Measurement of spinal flexion using the modified Schober Index (*see* p. 13) may help to monitor progression.

There are several techniques for eliciting sacroiliac tenderness but none is a wholly reliable test of sacroiliitis (*see* Chapter 1). If spinal involvement becomes extensive, the diagnosis may be suggested by a patient's posture and gait. A dorsal kyphosis may develop and walking is performed without the normal tilting of the pelvis. Cervical spine rotation may be limited so that attempts to look behind are achieved by rotation of the whole trunk. Chest movement is restricted at an early stage by involvement of costovertebral joints. Hip, knee or other peripheral joint involvement is characterized by the same signs seen in rheumatoid arthritis. Plantar fasciitis may be associated with heel tenderness.

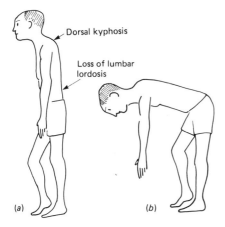

Figure 8.1 Posture of a man with severe ankylosing spondylitis. (a) The right leg is held in flexion due to hip involvement; and (b) on attempted spinal flexion, movement takes place mainly at the hips

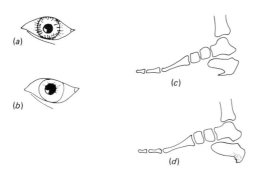

Figure 8.2 Ankylosing spondylitis. Anterior uveitis showing (a) active iritis, and (b) subsequent scarring of the iris. (c) Well delineated calcaneal spur often seen in asymptomatic subjects and in plantar fasciitis due to trauma. (d) Erosion of the calcaneum with poorly defined spur formation more typical of ankylosing spondylitis and other spondylarthropathies

Iritis occurs at some time in 30% and is marked by painful inflammation around the iris (*Figure 8.2(a)*). There may be pus in the anterior chamber. Residual scar tissue (synechiae) may tether the iris to the cornea, causing an irregular pupil (*Figure 8.2(b)*).

In severe, long-standing disease an aortitis may develop, giving rise to aortic regurgitation. Very rarely, other heart valves may become involved.

Differential diagnosis

The majority of patients present with low back pain, the causes of which are discussed in Chapter 6.

The development of painful dorsal kyphosis in a young person may be due to Scheuermann's disease.

The most discriminatory finding is the radiological demonstration of bilateral sacroiliitis. This may occasionally be confused with osteitis condensans ilii, an entity represented by painless sclerosis of the iliac side of the joint. In children and teenagers, the radiological appearance of the sacroiliac joints is indistinguishable from that of sacroiliitis in the adult. The radiological appearance of diffuse idiopathic skeletal hyperostosis may resemble that of ankylosing spondylitis. However, the intervertebral discs are uninvolved and there is no sacroiliitis.

Investigation

The investigation of persistent spinal pain is discussed in Chapter 6. An elevated ESR is usual in active spondylitis and is highest in those with peripheral arthritis. A mild anaemia may accompany the high ESR. Acute phase proteins such as CRP also rise sharply with peripheral joint involvement. Biochemistry is usually normal except occasional mild liver dysfunction. Tests for IgM RF are negative.

Sacroiliitis can be best detected by AP radiography of the pelvis. Oblique views usually offer no advantage. In early disease the sacroiliac joint margins become indistinct and this is followed by erosion and sclerosis of juxta-articular bone (*Figure 8.3*). Ankylosis and complete disappearance of the joints occur in late disease.

Early sacroiliitis may be difficult to determine. Technetium bone scans of the sacroiliac joints can be quantified and a high index suggests sacroiliitis. Anti-inflammatory drugs may reduce this to normal. CT scans of the sacroiliac joints can also provide useful evidence of disease at this site.

In the spine, the earliest change may be seen at the vertebral rims where small erosions occur (Romanus lesions). Syndesmophytes extend vertically from the vertebral margins and are

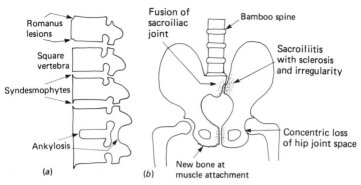

Figure 8.3   (a) Sequential stages of spinal ankylosis. (b) Sacroiliitis, inflammation of the symphysis pubis, ragged new bone at muscle attachments, hip involvement and advanced spinal ankylosis

often observed first at the dorsolumbar junction (*Figure 8.3(a)*). If the disease progresses, the syndesmophytes bridge the intervertebral space. Ossification of the whole intervertebral disc gives rise to the classical bamboo spine (*Figure 8.3(b)*). In a minority of cases a destructive discitis occurs. This resembles spinal infection but is distinguished by its presence at several levels. Erosions and sclerosis may occur at the symphysis pubis and tufts of new bone may arise around the pubis and iliac crests at the attachments of ligaments and muscle. Erosive calcaneal spurs are more indicative of plantar fasciitis than the prominent bone spurs seen in many healthy individuals (*Figure 8.2(c)* and *(d)*).

Peripheral arthritis of hips and knees may lead to loss of joint space but erosions are infrequent. Joint narrowing and erosion may occur in the hands and feet of a few patients and may resemble RA. Synovial fluid from inflamed peripheral joints is inflammatory in nature and identical to that seen in RA.

Chest radiographs sometimes reveal pulmonary apical fibrosis which is usually asymptomatic. Electrocardiographs show conduction defects in up to 10% of patients. These are more common than clinical valve disease and complete heart block may be a feature.

Aetiology

The finding of HLA B27 in 95% of patients with idiopathic ankylosing spondylitis points emphatically to a genetic predisposition. However, fewer than 5% of people with this antigen develop spondylitis, suggesting that other factors are equally important.

The spondylitis of reactive arthritis, inflammatory bowel disease and psoriatic arthritis is usually associated with HLA B27. In reactive arthritis, several organisms are known to precipitate the illness and an hypothesis which evokes infection as a cause of idiopathic ankylosing spondylitis is inescapable.

Serum immunoglobulin levels may be diffusely elevated in active disease but both serum and salivary IgA may be preferentially increased. This may indicate a mucosal response to foreign antigen in the gastrointestinal tract.

Although controversial, the isolation of *Klebsiella* organism from faeces and increased levels of specific anti-*Klebsiella* IgA suggest a role for this pathogen. It has been postulated that *Klebsiella* possesses antigens which are similar to HLA B27 and that cross-reacting antibodies initiate the disease. An alternative hypothesis involves the transfer of antigen from a *Klebsiella*-linked plasmid to B27 cells. Some patients with apparent idiopathic spondylitis may have unrecognized inflammatory bowel disease. A high proportion of all patients have deposits of IgG in the lamina propria of rectal mucosa but the significance of this is unknown.

Ankylosing spondylitis affects men more than women but the reason for this is uncertain. It is a milder disorder in women and probably goes unrecognized in many. The male to female ratio is approximately 4:1.

Pathology

Two major pathological processes can be identified:

1. an inflammatory enthesopathy, and
2. a synovitis of diarthrodial joints.

The former occurs at the site of ligament and joint capsule attachment to bone. The enthesopathy is associated with focal erosions which are replaced by bone as inflammation regresses. The process of ossification then extends from these sites. Romanus lesions on the vertebral bodies represent the erosive phase of syndesmophyte formation and occur where fibres of the annulus fibrosus are attached. This process may eventually involve the whole intervertebral disc. Inflammatory change at the sacroiliac and apophyseal joints is followed by ossification and joint fusion. The inflamed synovium of peripheral joints resembles RA microscopically and contains a similar array of lymphocytes. Aortic disease is characterized by inflammation and fibrosis of the aortic wall and subsequent dilatation of the aortic ring. The coronary vessels are not affected.

Treatment

Spinal pain and stiffness are often dramatically relieved by indomethacin or phenylbutazone. Some patients require small or only occasional doses. Other anti-inflammatory drugs tend to be less effective but are of value if the first choice drugs are precluded because of intolerance.

It is known that immobilization encourages ankylosis and it is likely that regular spinal exercises reduce this risk. Patients should be advised to perform their exercise programme once or twice daily. Instruction and encouragement by physiotherapists may be helpful. Some patients benefit from occasional periods of hydrotherapy.

When anti-inflammatory drugs are, for some reason, prohibited or when a patient is unresponsive to them, radiotherapy may be justified. Given in low dose to the spine and sacroiliac joints, it may abolish symptoms. There is a slightly increased risk of subsequent leukaemia or other malignant disease. It is inappropriate treatment for women who are still fertile.

Peripheral arthritis may improve with rest, splints and intra-articular corticosteroid injections.

Surgery has a limited role. Persistent knee inflammation may be treated by synovectomy but the results are less satisfactory than in RA. Hip and knee joint replacement are undertaken if necessary. There is a high risk of prosthetic joints ankylosing during the months following surgery. This may be lessened by prophylactic disodium etidronate. Spinal surgery is occasionally warranted to correct severe deformities which are incapacitating.

Course

Some patients have sacroiliitis and little or no spinal changes but others develop a bamboo spine. Disability is relatively mild and although 50% may be inconvenienced, and some may have to modify their work, loss of independence is rare.

Hip involvement has the most significant effect on mobility and handicap. Fracture of a rigid spine may occur after trauma and spinal cord compression is an uncommon but well documented complication. Severe and persistent disease activity may be associated with the development of amyloidosis.

Psoriatic arthropathy

Arthritis occurs in less than 10% of patients with psoriasis. Four broad patterns of joint inflammation occur:

1. Asymmetrical involvement of a small number of joints (70%);
2. Polyarthritis resembling RA, sometimes with prominent distal interphalangeal (DIP) joint inflammation;
3. A severely destructive polyarthritis (arthritis mutilans);
4. Ankylosing spondylitis.

Symptoms

Asymmetrical oligo-articular disease may begin abruptly with pain, stiffness and swelling of one or a few joints. A traumatic aetiology may be suspected and when the knee is involved patients may initially undergo investigation for a suspected orthopaedic disorder. The onset, character and distribution of joint symptoms may be identical to RA except that, apart from tenosynovitis, extra-articular features are rare. Heel pain due to plantar fasciitis may occur. Arthritis mutilans is a well known but uncommon outcome. Pain and stiffness may accompany profound disability in these cases. Sacroiliac and spinal involvement are characterized by the symptoms of ankylosing spondylitis. The severity of joint disease does not correlate with the activity or extent of the psoriasis.

Signs

In oligo-articular disease inflammation affects large or small joints asymmetrically. Involved digits may be sausage-shaped. The distribution of joint involvement may be indistinguishable from RA with symmetrical arthritis of small and large joints.

Prominent distal interphalangeal joint swelling is more common in psoriatic than rheumatoid arthritis. There is a correlation between this feature and psoriatic nail changes (*Figure 8.4(a)* and *(b)*). Arthritis mutilans is associated with gross deformities of fingers and other joints. Loss of bone may cause digital shortening, redundant soft tissues and so-called opera glass fingers (*Figure 8.4(d)*).

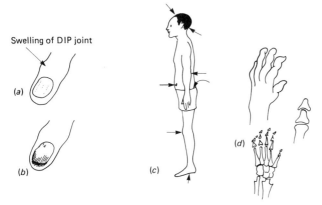

Swelling of DIP joint

(a)

(b)

(c)

(d)

Figure 8.4   Psoriatic arthropathy. Distal interphalangeal joint inflammation with (a) pitting of nails; (b) ridging and hyperkeratosis of nails (onycholysis); (c) sites to look for evidence of psoriasis; (d) arthritis mutilans showing hand deformity and severely destructive hand erosions as seen on a radiograph. A pencil in cup deformity of a distal interphalangeal joint is shown in more detail

Spinal involvement produces a clinical picture which is identical to that of idiopathic ankylosing spondylitis. Sacroiliitis and spondylitis may be apparent in association with any of the above patterns of peripheral joint disease.

There are several clinical variants of psoriasis, any of which may be associated with arthritis. The rash may be florid or concealed and patients may be unaware of any skin blemish. Inspection of likely sites of involvement such as the hair line, anal cleft and umbilicus may be rewarding when a patient has arthritis of obscure aetiology (*Figure 8.4(c)*). Finger and toe nails may be pitted, ridged or pushed away from the nail bed by hyperkeratosis (onycholysis).

Nodules, vasculitis, eye inflammation, peripheral neuropathy and internal organ involvement are not features of psoriatic arthropathy.

Differential diagnosis

Early oligo-articular disease involving a knee may resemble mechanical derangement. An acute onset may suggest gout, especially when a big toe joint is initially affected.

Distinction of the symmetrical pattern of disease from RA is difficult. The absence of extra-articular features and serum IgM rheumatoid factor (RF) may also be consistent with coincidental seronegative RA and psoriasis. Prominent distal interphalangeal joint involvement may resemble the Heberden nodes of generalized osteoarthritis. When active inflammation is confined to one or a few fingers, the swelling may look like tophaceous gout. Persistent reactive arthritis (Reiter's syndrome) may share several features of psoriatic arthritis. The asymmetrical distribution of arthritis, sausage swelling of digits, sacroiliitis and spondylitis, nail deformities and a rash resembling pustular psoriasis (keratodermia blenorrhagica) can make distinction impossible. The sacroiliitis of both psoriatic arthritis and Reiter's syndrome is sometimes unilateral whereas in idiopathic ankylosing spondylitis it is usually bilateral. Polyarthritis associated with other rashes may cause confusion. Pityriasis and eczema, especially when the latter involves the nails, can resemble psoriasis. Psoriatic nail involvement may be difficult to distinguish from fungal infection. Minor nail pitting can occur in healthy individuals. Caution is therefore required before attributing joint symptoms to psoriatic arthropathy when the only manifestation of cutaneous disease is abnormal nails.

Investigations

Active disease is associated with elevation of ESR, acute phase proteins and immunoglobulins. Anaemia accompanying these changes may have the same characteristics of that seen in RA. IgM rheumatoid factor occurs with no greater frequency than that of the healthy population. Synovial fluid analysis reveals inflammatory levels of polymorphs but there are no other distinctive features. It has been claimed that hyperuricaemia may accompany psoriasis and psoriatic arthritis but recent studies have failed to confirm this.

Radiographs may show a spectrum of change from loss of joint space to severe destruction and bone lysis. Erosions may be identical to those of RA. In arthritis mutilans, there may be extensive loss of juxta-articular bone and so-called pencil in cup deformities (*Figure 8.4(d)*). These changes are occasionally seen in RA and are not exclusive to psoriatic arthropathy.

Resorption of the terminal tuft is a feature. It also occurs in scleroderma and hyperparathyroidism but is not seen in RA. The appearance of the sacroiliitis is the same as that of idiopathic ankylosing spondylitis except that it is more likely to be unilateral. Syndesmophytes on the vertebral bodies may be identical to those of ankylosing spondylitis but sometimes they are thicker and appear to be attached to the middle of the vertebrae rather than their margins. Even less commonly, there may be distinctive paravertebral ossification. Ragged new bone at muscle attachments and erosive or fluffy calcaneal spurs are findings which are also seen in idiopathic ankylosing spondylitis.

Aetiology

Unlike RA there is an almost equal sex distribution. The exact relationship between psoriasis and arthritis is obscure because the severity of one does not predictably influence that of the other.

There is a familial association of both psoriasis and psoriatic arthropathy and an undoubted genetic contribution to both. Psoriasis occurs in about 6% of the population and is associated with HLA B13 and HLA B17. Psoriatic peripheral arthritis has been linked to HLA DR7. Susceptibility to psoriatic spondylitis is increased by the presence of HLA B27 but this antigen is found in 60–80% of patients compared with more than 95% in idiopathic ankylosing spondylitis.

Although IgA and IgG rheumatoid factors may be demonstrated their aetiological significance is uncertain. Immune complexes occur in about 60% but these are also seen in uncomplicated psoriasis and the levels are lower than in RA. Evidence of complement activation is only rarely found.

Pathology

Peripheral arthritis is associated with synovial changes which are indistinguishable from those of RA. Synovial hypertrophy, lymphocyte infiltration and both erosion and uniform loss of cartilage are all features. Granulomata are absent and vasculitis does not occur. The histopathology of the sacroiliitis and spondylitis is identical to that of ankylosing spondylitis.

Treatment

Management is dictated by the distribution of joint involvement. The peripheral arthritis is treated in almost the same way as that of RA. Rest, splints, intra-articular corticosteroids, anti-inflammatory drugs, and analgesics provide a therapeutic basis.

Second-line treatment of severe or progressive disease with sodium aurothiomalate is effective but D-penicillamine is not known to be helpful. Antimalarials are inadvisable because they may cause severe worsening of psoriasis. Immunosuppressive agents have been used successfully to treat both the skin and joint disease. Azathioprine and methotrexate are of proven value. The retinoid preparation, etretinate, is effective for socially disabling psoriasis and may also lessen joint inflammation. Its use is hampered by toxicity. It is unlikely that second-line treatments influence sacroiliitis or spondylitis, the treatment of which is that described for ankylosing spondylitis.

The indications for surgery are the same as for RA but the need for orthopaedic intervention is less frequent.

Course

In general, psoriatic arthropathy causes less disability than RA. A small percentage with arthritis mutilans or severe spondylitis may lose some measure of independence.

Reactive arthritis (Reiter's syndrome)

This constitutes a variable syndrome of arthritis, eye inflammation and mucocutaneous lesions. It follows specific infections in genetically susceptible individuals.

Symptoms

The presenting symptoms are invariably acute. Within a few days or weeks of an infectious enteritis or non-specific urethritis, arthralgia, fever and painful swelling of one or a few joints may develop. Initially knees or ankles are more likely to be involved but there may be small joint swelling as well as spinal pain. Painful mouth ulcers occur and these are occasionally distressing. Redness and soreness of an eye may precede or accompany joint symptoms but is not seen in all cases. Plantar fasciitis and Achilles tendonitis are common at some stage in the evolution of the disease.

Some of those with a history of recent enteritis may subsequently develop symptoms of urethritis (frequency, dysuria and urethral discharge). Other patients presenting with arthritis may have no recollection of an infectious illness. Although often considered a self-limiting disease, at least 60% of patients develop intermittent or chronic joint symptoms. Low back pain and stiffness may worsen in 30% due to persistent sacroiliitis and progressive spondylitis.

Signs

Asymmetrical large joint inflammation is characteristic. Small joint involvement may lead to sausage-shaped digits similar to those of psoriatic arthritis (*Figure 8.5(a)*). Initial spinal tenderness may be followed over months or years by the unmistakable picture of ankylosing spondylitis. Eye inflammation is usually that of conjuctivitis but iritis may occur, especially in the chronic disease.

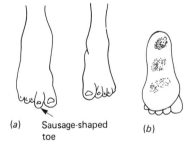

(a)   Sausage-shaped toe   (b)

Figure 8.5 Reactive arthritis. (a) Asymmetrical polyarthritis with considerable swelling of the involved ankle and a sausage-shaped toe; (b) keratodermia blenorrhagica on the soles

Nail changes similar to those of psoriasis may develop and a rash, keratodermia blenorrhagica, may affect the soles of the feet (*Figure 8.5(b)*). This is virtually indistinguishable from pustular psoriasis. When the precipitating organism is *Yersinia enterocolitica*, the acute illness may also be associated with erythema nodosum. When aphthous ulcers are present in the mouth or pharynx, they have no special characteristics. Discharge from the penis may be asymptomatic and although circinate balanitis may be a recurrent feature, it is often ignored by patients. It should always be sought by examiners.

Differential diagnosis

Symptoms confined to one or a few joints in the presence of persistent bacterial infection may suggest septic arthritis. A history of urethritis requires exclusion of gonococcal septic arthritis by blood, synovial fluid and urethral culture. Other causes of acute arthritis, such as gout and pseudogout, can be investigated by examination of synovial fluid for crystals (*see* Chapter 11).

Symptoms of enteritis usually resolve but occasionally loose stools persist. The arthritis of inflammatory bowel disease may then need to be considered as well as Whipple's disease, a rare enteropathic cause of arthritis (*see* p. 96).

In the presence of nail deformities or keratoderma blenorrhagica, chronic reactive arthritis may be impossible to distinguish from psoriatic arthropathy.

Buccal ulceration, arthritis and iritis are regular findings in Behcet's syndrome. However, other features of this illness are not seen.

Investigations

Clinical evidence of continuing infection should be pursued. Blood and stool culture for *Salmonella, Shigella* or *Yersinia* organisms may be rewarding. Circulating antibody levels may reveal evidence of recent infection by one of these agents. Cultures of a urethral discharge may occasionally yield evidence of *Chlamydia* infection but usually they are sterile.

Elevation of ESR and other acute phase proteins may be accompanied by a diffuse increase of immunoglobulins. IgM rheumatoid factor is absent.

The synovial fluid usually contains large numbers of polymorph leukocytes. So-called Reiter's cells (Pekin cells) are synovial fluid monocytes containing polymorphs. They may be seen in reactive arthritis but can occur in several other joint diseases and are not a specific finding. Tissue typing is justifiable in the absence of a typical clinical picture. The presence of HLA B27 provides circumstantial evidence in favour of the diagnosis.

Radiological signs may include occasional erosions of peripheral joints, sacroiliitis which is sometimes unilateral, and all the features of ankylosing spondylitis.

Aetiology

The syndrome appears to affect men 10 times more frequently than women when precipitated by urethritis. This may simply reflect the difficulty of establishing genital infection in women because amongst those with an enteric aetiology the sex ratio is equal.

Chlamydia trachomatis infection can be incriminated in 30% of those with urethritis. *Shigella flexneri* (dysentery) and *Salmonella* species account for the majority with enteritis. *Yersina enterocolitica* occurs chiefly in Scandinavia but cases do arise in other parts of Europe and in N. America. Reactive arthritis has also been described following *Campylobacter jejuni* infection.

Amongst Caucasians with reactive arthritis, HLA B27 is found in 80%. In some other races this association does not apply.

Pathology

The pathology of the peripheral arthritis resembles that of RA and that of the spine is the same as in ankylosing spondylitis.

Treatment

If urethritis is a suspected cause, further exposure to infection must be discouraged. Care must be taken not to embarrass or antagonize patients whose urethritis follows enteritic reactive arthritis. There is little evidence that antibiotic treatment of urethritis modifies the arthritis. The tenets of treatment are those of any peripheral arthritis. Intra-articular injections of corticosteroid and oral anti-inflammatory drugs tend to be less effective than in other inflammatory joint disorders. For those with spinal involvement, the management is that described for ankylosing spondylitis.

Course

Reactive arthritis is notoriously difficult to treat when it follows a chronic course. Spontaneous remissions and relapses are characteristic. Sodium aurothiomalate, D-penicillamine and other second-line drugs have no acknowledged effect. Some disability occurs in 40% and, in general, the outcome is worse than in psoriatic arthropathy.

Enteropathic arthritis

In addition to the peripheral and spinal disease of reactive arthritis there are other associations of bowel and joint disease.

Inflammatory bowel disease

Peripheral arthritis complicates approximately 15% of patients with ulcerative colitis and Crohn's disease. Inflammation affects predominantly large joints and tends to fluctuate with the activity of the bowel symptoms. There is no consistent association of arthritis with other systemic features of inflammatory bowel disease such as erythema nodosum and iritis. There is no link with any specific HLA type. Deformity and cartilage destruction are not features of this arthritis.

A further 5% of patients may develop the clinical and radiological picture of ankylosing spondylitis. The spinal disease sometimes precedes evidence of bowel inflammation. Approximately 70% of such patients possess HLA B27 and the spondylitis pursues a course independent of bowel inflammation. Radiological evidence of sacroiliitis occurs without symptoms in some cases, often unassociated with HLA B27.

Treatment of both spinal and peripheral joint disease involves the use of conventional anti-inflammatory drugs. These can be prescribed without fear of worsening the bowel symptoms.

Total colectomy in ulcerative colitis and large bowel Crohn's disease may abolish the peripheral arthritis but does not influence established ankylosing spondylitis.

Intestinal bypass arthritis

Arthralgia and arthritis may accompany 10% of patients who have undergone jejunocolic bypass surgery for morbid obesity. Knees, ankles and fingers are affected with equal frequency and the symptoms tend to be episodic although some cases develop persistent joint swelling. Spinal pain is common but true sacroiliitis and spondylitis do not seem to be features. Associated symptoms include cutaneous vasculitis and erythema nodosum.

The disease may be mediated by circulating immune complexes which are formed in response to bacterial overgrowth of blind loops of bowel. There is no HLA association.

Treatment comprises analgesics and anti-inflammatory drugs, antibiotics to alter gut flora and, if necessary, reconstitution of the bowel lumen.

Whipple's disease

This is a rare disorder which affects mainly men. The principal features are transient episodes of large joint arthritis, diarrhoea, lymph node enlargement and fever. Pigmentation, weight loss and other evidence of malabsorption are secondary to steatorrhoea.

The diagnosis is established by demonstrating the presence of PAS staining 'foamy' macrophages in the villi of jejunal biopsy samples. Similar inclusions have been demonstrated in synovium, lymph nodes and other sites.

Prolonged treatment with broad spectrum antibiotics usually eradicates the symptoms which can otherwise prove fatal.

Further reading

CAMERON, F. *et al.* (1983). Is a *Klebsiella* plasmid involved in the aetiology of ankylosing spondylitis in HLA B27 positive individuals? *Mol. Immunol.* **20**, 563

CARETTE, S. *et al.* (1983). The natural disease cause of ankylosing spondylitis. *Arthritis Rheum.*, **26**, 186

ENLOW, R. *et al.* (1980). The spondylitis of inflammatory bowel disease – evidence for a non HLA-linked axial arthropathy. *Arthritis Rheum.*, **23**, 1359

LEIRISALO, M. *et al.* (1982). Follow up study on patients with Reiter's disease and reactive arthritis with special reference to HLA B27. *Arthritis Rheum.*, **25**, 249

van ROMUNDE, L. *et al.* (1984). Psoriasis and arthritis. *Rheum. Int.* **4**, 55

YLI-KERTTULA, U. (1984). Clinical characterisation in male and female uro-arthritis or Reiter's syndrome. *Clin. Rheum.*, **3**, 351

9
Behçet's syndrome

This is a rare disorder in Europe and America and is more common in Japan and some Middle Eastern countries.

Symptoms

The illness usually begins insidiously with oral or genital ulcers. Painful swelling of large joints or arthralgia occurs in 60%. Spinal pain may be a feature but stiffness is not prominent. These complaints may develop simultaneously or in succession over a variable period, and they tend to become recurrent. Fever, painful skin lesions, headache and neurological symptoms may develop in the course of the disease. Eye inflammation and visual impairment usually occur when the illness has been established for several years.

Signs

Buccal ulceration is painful and takes the form of minor or major aphthous lesions, sometimes involving the oropharynx. Genital ulcers occur over the scrotum and penis or in the vagina. These look worse than they feel and patients do not always volunteer their presence.

Inflammation of knees, ankles and less commonly of wrists or smaller joints may be accompanied by other features. The most common skin manifestation is erythema nodosum. Superficial thrombophlebitis also occurs in some patients. Other skin lesions include pustules and papules. The central nervous system may be involved, usually as a late manifestation. Meningitis, stroke syndromes and cerebellar signs have all been recorded. Thrombosis of calf veins and other vessels including major arteries may occur. Iritis may be the outward evidence of a pan-uveitis which affects more than 50%. Examination of the retina by fluorescence may show evidence of vasculitis.

Differential diagnosis

There are no specific laboratory characteristics and the diagnosis must be established clinically. Oral ulceration, arthritis and iritis may suggest reactive arthritis, and distinction may not be possible in the absence of additional signs. Sacroiliitis and spondylitis do not occur in Behçet's syndrome, despite frequent spinal pain. There is no relationship with HLA B27.

Arthritis, erythema nodosum and eye inflammation may arouse suspicion of inflammatory bowel disease or sarcoidosis. Bowel studies or biopsy for evidence of sarcoid granuloma may be warranted.

Central nervous system involvement, thrombosis and arthritis may superficially resemble systemic lupus erythematosus (SLE) or polyarteritis nodosa (PAN). However, intermittent large joint arthritis is not usual in SLE or PAN and serological characteristics of SLE do not occur.

The pathergy test involves pricking the skin with a sterile needle. When positive, pustules develop at the sites of injury. In Turkey, where Behçet's syndrome is common, this is a reliable diagnostic test for the disease, but in Britain, where it is rare, it has for some reason no discriminatory value.

Investigations

During active phases of the disease a high ESR and mild hypochromic anaemia are common. A diffuse increase of immunoglobulins is usual. Rheumatoid factors, autoantibodies and alterations of serum complement are not found. Examination of synovial fluid reveals an inflammatory effusion, the leukocyte count sometimes approaching that of septic arthritis.

There are no specific radiological features and although some loss of cartilage may occur after years of recurrent episodes of arthritis, joint erosions are rare.

Where neurological involvement has occurred, CSF examination shows a modest number of lymphocytes but little or no rise in proteins.

Venography or arteriography may be necessary to determine the presence and extent of thrombosis.

Aetiology

The striking geographical distribution may reflect both environmental and genetic factors. In Japan, the prevalence is such that Behçet's syndrome is amongst the most common cause of blindness. Men are affected more frequently than women. In the Japanese and Turkish populations there is an association with HLA B5 and DR5.

Circulating immune complexes, increased motility of polymorphs and diminished helper T cell populations are amongst the immunological abnormalities which have been observed.

Pathology

The ulcers are associated with non-specific chronic inflammation. Synovium is occasionally replaced by granulation tissue but more often the changes resemble those of RA and other inflammatory disorders.

Treatment

The oral ulcers may respond to locally applied pastes and corticosteroids. Management of the arthritis involves anti-inflammatory drugs, joint aspiration and, when necessary, intra-articular corticosteroids. Severe eye or neurological disease warrants treatment with oral corticosteroids or immunosuppressive agents, of which chlorambucil appears the most effective.

Course

The prognosis varies with the disease severity. Treatment may halt the progression of eye disease and improve mild neurological symptoms. Blindness and serious neurological sequelae may occur despite the best endeavours. Disability rather than death is the outcome in the minority of patients with severe disease.

Further reading

CHAJEK, T. and FAINARU, M. (1975). Behçet's disease. Report of 41 cases and a review of the literature. *Medicine,* **54,** 179

LEHNER, T. *et al.* (1982). The relationship of HLA B and DR phenotypes to Behçet's syndrome, recurrent oral ulceration and the class of immune complexes. *Immunology,* **47,** 581

10
Polymyalgia rheumatica

This is a relatively common illness of elderly subjects. Its recognition is important because of its relationship with giant cell arteritis (cranial arteritis, temporal arteritis). It is likely that these entities represent the same disease process but polymyalgia is the more frequent manifestation.

Symptoms

Usually symptoms begin acutely with upper and lower limb girdle pain and stiffness, worse in the mornings. Less frequently the onset is insidious. Difficulty in dressing, washing and coping with stairs is usual. Weakness is a variable complaint but easy fatigue and lassitude are common.

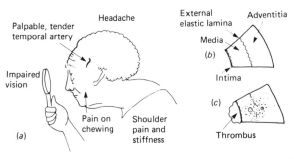

Figure 10.1 Polymyalgia rheumatica and cranial arteritis. (a) Clinical features; (b) section of a normal artery; (c) involved artery showing dense chronic inflammatory cell infiltration with two giant cells, fragmentation of the external elastic lamina, and thrombus formation on the intima

Headache, visual disturbance or blindness are the symptomatic hallmarks of giant cell arteritis and these may occur in the absence of musculoskeletal symptoms. However, they may also appear within weeks or even years after the onset of muscle discomfort. Pain in the face or jaw on chewing is another feature of the arteritis when it affects vessels of the head (*Figure 10.1(a)*).

Signs

Polymyalgia is characterized by a paucity of signs. There may be tenderness of the shoulders and sternoclavicular joints and shoulder movement may be slightly impaired. Evidence of wasting or weakness is absent. Swelling of the sternoclavicular joints and small effusions of the knees or other joints may be observed but these are transient. Tenderness of the scalp or cranial arteries is rarely found in the absence of symptoms affecting the head or face. When headache or blurred vision are features it is common to find tenderness and thickening of one or both cranial arteries. Fundoscopy may reveal swelling or palor of the optic disc with occasional exudates and haemorrhages. Auscultation for bruits may rarely provide evidence of large vessel arteritis.

Differential diagnosis

The clinical picture of proximal muscle pain and stiffness associated with a very high ESR in an elderly person is virtually diagnostic. Bone pain and similar elevation of ESR may occur in metastatic malignant disease or myelomatosis. Radiographs, bone scans or marrow aspiration may be required to rule out malignancy.

In the elderly, RA may present with a clinical picture similar to polymyalgia rheumatica. The ESR tends to be moderately elevated and the presence of a high titre of IgM RF may suggest the correct diagnosis. Peripheral synovitis may occur in both disorders but persistent joint swelling or subsequent deformities are consistent only with RA.

Cervical spondylosis and adhesive capsulitis of the shoulders can usually be excluded on clinical grounds. These are associated with painful restriction of the neck or pronounced impairment of shoulder movement.

Muscle pain caused by hypothyroidism or calcium disorders should be distinguished by their concomitant clinical or laboratory features. A very high ESR is found in neither condition.

Polymyositis is associated with weakness and, later, wasting. These are not features of polymyalgia. Muscle enzymes and electromyography are abnormal in myositis.

Giant cell arteritis is unlike any other pattern of vasculitis in its distribution and should not be confused with polyarteritis nodosa or other rarer patterns of vasculitis.

Investigations

A very high ESR (usually $>60\,\mathrm{mm\,h^{-1}}$) which falls rapidly during treatment is characteristic. This may be accompanied by mild anaemia and liver dysfunction. Muscle enzyme levels and electromyography are normal.

Radiographs of joints are also normal but erosions of the sternoclavicular joints have been described. Technetium bone scans may reveal abnormal uptake at juxta-articular bone sites.

Temporal artery biopsy is indicated whenever giant cell arteritis is suspected clincially. The majority of patients with polymyalgia do not have scalp tenderness but temporal artery biopsy will reveal evidence of giant cell arteritis in at least 30% and there is a good argument for performing this investigation in all patients whether or not they have clinical arteritis. Although it may not influence treatment, it may establish the diagnosis beyond question. The changes in the temporal artery may be localized and sampling errors are common. Corticosteroids diminish the chances of positive biopsy within days of beginning treatment.

Aetiology

The disease is rare below the age of 50 and begins most commonly beyond the age of 70. It is twice as common in females and is rare in non-Caucasians. There is a weak association with HLA DR4. Elevated levels of circulating immune complexes are seen in active disease but complement levels are unaltered. Reduced numbers of circulating suppressor T cells have been observed.

Pathology

Although symptoms suggest that polymyalgia is a myopathic disease, no pathological features occur in muscles. There is some evidence of proximal joint synovitis as manifest by abnormal bone scans, arthroscopic inflammation and microscopic inflammatory cell infiltrates.

At involved sites in the temporal arteries, all layers of the vessel wall may be densely infiltrated with lymphocytes, histiocytes and multinucleate giant cells (see Figure 10.1(b) and (c)). The elastic laminae and the elastic fibres of the media may be disrupted and thrombi may occlude the lumen. Fibrinoid changes do not occur but deposits of immunoglobulin and complement are found in the arterial wall. Similar lesions may be found in the aorta, carotid, ophthalmic and posterior ciliary vessels. It is involvement of the latter which causes visual impairment. The ophthalmic artery is usually spared.

Treatment

Once the clinical diagnosis is suspected it is advisable to begin treatment with corticosteroids, delaying only if a temporal artery biopsy is planned. The dose of steroid is arbitrary but it is wiser to employ an initially large dose (e.g. prednisolone 60 mg) when giant cell arteritis is clinically apparent. In polymyalgia without symptoms or signs of cranial vessel disease, one-third of this dose is usually adequate. The corticosteroids should be reduced over a period of weeks to a dose compatible with symptomatic relief.

Non-steroidal anti-inflammatory drugs also reduce polymyalgic symptoms but steroids are preferable because of the ophthalmic risks associated with occult vasculitis.

Treatment has to be continued for at least a year.

Course

Polymyalgia rheumatica responds dramatically to corticosteroids. If pain and stiffness do not improve within days, the diagnosis is probably mistaken.

Deterioration of sight may be averted by treatment but once blindness occurs it is irreversible.

The disease is self-limiting and usually resolves over 1–5 years. A minority of patients require life-long treatment.

Occasionally, aortic involvement may result in a dissecting aneurysm. Myocardial infarction and neurological symptoms are rare complications of the vasculitis.

Further reading

ARMSTRONG, R. et al. (1983). Histocompatibility antigens in polymyalgia rheumatica and giant cell arteritis. J. Rheum., **10,** 659

BENGTSSON, B. and MALMWELL, B. (1981). The epidemiology of giant cell arteritis including temporal arteritis and polymyalgia rheumatica. Incidence of different clinical presentations and eye complications. Arthritis Rheum., **24,** 899

11
Acute arthritis

Investigation of acute arthritis

Acute joint pain may be associated with severe discomfort and demand urgent investigation. Acute arthritis often involves a single joint but investigation of any monoarthritis requires the same diagnostic approach. The possible causes are:

1. Trauma;
2. Gout;
3. Pseudogout;
4. Infection;
5. Acute or monoarticular onset of polyarthrits.

TABLE 11.1   Synovial fluid characteristics

	Appear-ance	Viscosity	Leukocyte count $(\times 10^9 \, l^{-1})$	Predominant cell	Stain or wet preparation
Trauma	1. Clear 2. Blood	High	<2.0	Mononuclear	–
Osteoarthritis	Clear	High	<2.0	Mononuclear	Cartilage fragments
Gout	Turbid-purulent	Low	2.0–50	Polymorph	Monosodium urate crystals
Pseudogout	Turbid-purulent	Low	2.0–50	Polymorph	Calcium pyrophosphate crystals
Rheumatoid arthritis	Turbid	Low	>2.0	Polymorph	–
Sepsis	Purulent	Low	>50	Polymorph	Bacteria
Tuberculosis	Turbid	Low	>2.0	Polymorph	Usually no organisms

The clinical context may give some indication of the most likely diagnosis. Examination of synovial fluid is the single most important investigation (*see Table 11.1*). Demonstration of hyperuricaemia, cartilage calcification (chondrocalcinosis) or other abnormalities may provide additional diagnostic information but may also be misleading.

Trauma

If symptoms occur after an obvious injury, further investigation may depend on the outcome of rest and other symptomatic measures.

In young athletic subjects, sprains and twisting injuries of a knee or ankle are common but if no clear episode of trauma can be recalled it is prudent to consider the alternative possibilities. The onset of diseases such as gout, reactive arthritis and ankylosing spondylitis is often wrongly attributed to trauma in young people.

A history of knee injury without an obvious collateral ligament tear but which is followed by persistent pain, recurrent effusions or locking, is most likely due to a meniscal or anterior cruciate ligament tear. Further investigation may involve examination of synovial fluid, arthrography and arthroscopy.

Synovial fluid may be densely blood-stained after recent trauma and this is common in elderly patients who have fallen. The fluid may also be xanthochromic or clear with a high viscosity and a low cell count.

Arthrograms involve the injection of contrast material and air into a joint to allow definition of internal structures by radiography. This technique may reveal torn menisci or other damage.

Arthroscopy allows direct visualization of the joint interior. Its best application is in the preoperative evaluation of suspected mechanical injury. It also allows inspection and biopsy of the synovium.

Gout, pseudogout and infection

These may all cause a hot swollen joint with fever and leukocytosis. The best means of discriminating between them is synovial fluid analysis.

In all three disorders the synovial fluid may be turbid or purulent and contain large numbers of leukocytes (*Figure 11.1*). It is therefore essential to examine all samples under a compensated polarizing microscope. Crystals of monosodium urate or calcium pyrophosphate will be apparent in gout or pseudogout respectively. The former are long, thin, needle-shaped and brightly birefringent. The latter are small, chunky or rhomboid in shape and weakly birefringent. The optical properties of the crystals are the opposite of each other, with birefringence being exhibited only when the axes of individual crystals are properly aligned (*Figure 11.1(a)* and *(b)*).

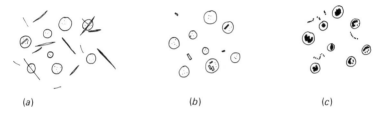

(a)   (b)   (c)

Figure 11.1 Synovial fluid in acute arthritis contains many polymorphs. (a) Monosodium urate crystals which are numerous, slender and mainly needle-shaped. (b) Calcium pyrophosphate crystals which are fewer, blunt or rhomboid in shape and have the opposite birefringent properties to monosodium urate. (c) Gram stain showing Gram-positive cocci in septic arthritis

Purulent or densely turbid fluid which contains no crystals should be presumed to be septic. Additional investigations should then include Gram staining and culture of the synovial fluid, blood cultures and swabs of the genital and oropharyngeal regions for gonococci in young, sexually active patients (*Figure 11.1(c)*).

Faintly turbid synovial fluid which contains no crystals is less likely to be septic but should nevertheless be cultured for both pyogenic organisms and tubercle bacilli. Tuberculous monoarthritis is not usually of acute onset but its exclusion is the principal reason for performing synovial biopsy. This should be undertaken if all other investigations of single joint arthritis have failed to yield a diagnosis.

Biopsy can be achieved with a special needle or through an arthroscope. If the hip joint is suspect, its inaccessiblity makes it best to obtain a surgical biopsy under a general anaesthetic. This is also the preferable technique for any biopsy undertaken in children.

Acute or monoarticular onset of polyarthritis

If synovial fluid analysis reveals no crystals, no organisms and the fluid is of low viscosity with an inflammatory leukocyte count, other investigations assume more importance.

A high ESR may confirm the inflammatory nature of the disorder. A positive test for IgM RF makes RA a likely diagnosis. The presence of hyperuricaemia may prompt further examination of synovial fluid for urate crystals but hyperuricaemia is common and does not always denote gout.

Radiographs of the hands and feet may reveal early asymptomatic erosions of RA or psoriatic arthropathy. Views of the pelvis may show unsuspected sacroiliitis suggesting one of the spondylarthritic diseases (see Chapter 8). Chondrocalcinosis of the involved joint may be coincidental but calcium pyrophosphate crystals are sometimes difficult to see and further synovial fluid analysis may be worthwhile.

Only when these possibilities have been pursued is synovial biopsy indicated but it must be remembered that in most diseases the range of synovial pathology is similar and non-specific. Biopsy is therefore hardly ever justifiable for the diagnosis of a polyarthritis.

Gout

This common cause of acute arthritis has a prevalence which correlates with the availability of plentiful food and drink.

Symptoms

The initial episode usually affects a first metatarsophalangeal joint (podagra). The joint becomes excruciatingly painful and swollen (*Figure 11.2(a)*). Similar symptoms may affect any synovial joint and

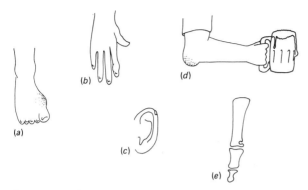

Figure 11.2 Gout. (a) Acute inflammation of the first metatarsophalangeal joint (podagra); (b) tophus on a distal interphalangeal joint; (c) tophus on ear; (d) olecranon bursitis due to gout; (e) typical gouty erosion with characteristic punched-out appearance

in subsequent attacks several sites may be involved simultaneously. Pain often begins at night or may be precipitated by illness, surgery or dietary excess.

Signs

The typical patient is an obese man who enjoys drinking alcohol, but postmenopausal women are also affected.

An involved joint is usually hot, red and shiny, often with extensive oedema. A whole hand or foot may become swollen when gout affects a single small joint. As the attack regresses the overlying skin may exfoliate. Fever is common. Recurrent episodes of acute gout affect increasing numbers of joints. The accumulation of monosodium urate crystals within and around toes and fingers leads to chronic swelling and deformity. Distal interphalangeal joints are favoured sites for tophaceous deposits (see Figure 11.2(b)).

Pale, creamy subcutaneous tophi may be seen on the pinnae, Achilles tendons or in olecranon bursae where they have a granular appearance (Figure 11.2(c) and (d)). Tophi may also occur at unusual sites such as the finger pulp. They sometimes ulcerate, especially during hypouricaemic treatment. Elderly patients may develop large tophi without exhibiting gout. These are often patients receiving diuretics.

Hypertension, a palpable liver and signs of hepatocellular disease may be apparent. Uric acid kidney stones are rarely seen in primary gout but acute renal failure may follow precipitation of crystals in the tubules during uricosuric treatment of gout and the increased excretion of uric acid which follows treatment of myeloproliferative diseases. Calcium stones are more common in subjects with hyperuricaemia, many of whom do not have gout.

Differential diagnosis

The other causes of acute arthritis are discussed in the preceding chapter. Swelling and erythema may be sufficiently intense to resemble infective cellulitis. Tophi in the distal interphalangeal joints may resemble Heberden nodes. The distal interphalangeal joint swelling of psoriatic arthritis and of reactive arthritis may also look like gout. Rarely, joint deformities may suggest the polyarticular picture of RA. This may be the more so if tophi occur on the elbows where they may resemble rheumatoid nodules.

Investigation

Demonstration of monosodium urate crystals in joint fluid or tophaceous material is the most certain way of establishing the diagnosis. Hyperuricaemia is usual and in patients with podagra or episodic joint inflammation it is presumptive evidence of gout. However, hyperuricaemia is a common asymptomatic finding and may co-exist with other joint disorders. Macrocytosis and biochemical evidence of liver dysfunction are not infrequent findings and imply alcohol abuse. Serum triglyceride levels are often raised for the same reason. In patients who are hypertensive, or receiving diuretics, elevation of blood urea or creatinine may be observed. During acute attacks a high ESR and peripheral leukocytosis are common. In chronic tophaceous gout radiographs may show small, well circumscribed erosions, loss of joint space and secondary osteoarthritis (*see Figure 11.2(e)*).

Aetiology

Uric acid is derived from purines produced in the liver or ingested in the diet. The blood level of uric acid is higher in men than women and this explains why gout is 20 times more frequent in males. After menopause, the blood uric acid of women rises and eventually matches that of men. A family history of gout is common, suggesting an inherited factor. Some indigenous people of the Pacific have a natural tendency to hyperuricaemia and up to 10% of New Zealand Maori men have gout.

The majority of patients with gout exhibit relatively poor excretion of uric acid. When exposed to dietary, drug or other hyperuricaemic risk factors, the effect on blood uric acid is magnified.

There is a close relationship between hyperuricaemia and obesity. The typical man with gout has a high energy diet, often due to the consumption of excessive alcohol. The purine intake of patients with gout is not usually remarkable.

Alcohol induces hyperuricaemia by three mechanisms:

1. Accentuation of purine turnover in the liver;
2. Absorption of purines contained in beer;
3. Impaired renal clearance of uric acid by lactic acid formed from ethanol.

In the kidney, uric acid is wholly filtered at the glomerulus, almost completely reabsorbed and then secreted in small quantities back into the proximal tubular lumen. It is at these sites of reabsorption and secretion that lactic acid and other chemicals exert their effect. Uric acid excretion may be impaired by the ketosis of fasting, small doses of aspirin, lead poisoning and diuretics. Paradoxically, large doses of aspirin increase uric acid excretion.

Very few patients with hyperuricaemia have a naturally high production of uric acid. Secondary gout may follow the rapid breakdown of purines during treatment of myeloproliferative diseases. Overproduction occurs in the very rare X-linked deficiency of hypoxanthine guanine phosphoribosyl transferase (HGPRT). This results in a failure of hypoxanthine reutilization and of the feedback inhibition of *de novo* purine synthesis (*Figure 11.3*). Complete deficiency of HGPRT results in a syndrome of juvenile gout, kidney stones, renal failure and brain damage (Lesch Nyhan syndrome). Partial deficiency is associated with gout and less severe neurological impairment.

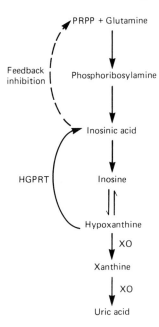

Figure 11.3 *De novo* production of uric acid. PRPP = phosphoribosyl pyrophosphate; XO = xanthine oxidase; HGPRT = hypoxanthine guanine phosphoribosyl transferase

Sustained hyperuricaemia leads to tophaceous deposits in cartilage and synovium. Abrupt reductions of blood urate levels such as may follow the introduction of treatment or the end of a drinking bout, disturb urate homeostasis. Dissolution of uric acid from tophi is followed by loosening and shedding of crystals. The presence of free crystals initiates an acute inflammatory response in which interleukin-1, acute phase proteins, complement and other mediators play a role. Phagocytosis of IgG coated crystals is an important step in this process but the exact sequence involved in the initiation and termination of an acute attack is unclear.

Pathology

Within the joint microtophi form in the synovium and articular cartilage. As these increase in size they may erode bone in the same fashion as the inflamed synovium of RA. Frequent episodes of inflammation may lead to loss of cartilage and secondary osteoarthritis.

Gouty nephropathy is rarely seen today but chronic, untreated gout may be associated with precipitation of crystals in the renal parenchyma. These cause inflammation, scarring and a gradual impairment of renal function. Crystals may also form in the tubules when large amounts of uric acid are excreted.

Treatment

Management of gout falls into two phases.

First, the acute arthritis is treated with indomethacin or other anti-inflammatory drugs. Colchicine may be used when anti-inflammatory agents are contraindicated, as in renal failure or peptic ulceration. Colchicine may cause abdominal pain and diarrhoea. Large joint involvement may respond to aspiration and intra-articular corticosteroid injection.

Secondly, persistent hyperuricaemia may be treated by weight reduction and limitation of alcohol intake but these are difficult to achieve. Diuretics should be withdrawn if possible. Hypo-uricaemic drugs should be used if these measures fail. Probenecid and sulphinpyrazone are uricosuric agents which act by blocking tubular reabsorption of uric acid. Patients should increase their fluid intake during the first few days of treatment to lessen the risk of crystal precipitation within the renal collecting ducts. Allo-purinol competitively inhibits xanthine oxidase, reducing the production of uric acid (*Figure 11.3*). This is the preparation of choice in renal failure or urate overproduction.

Hypouricaemic treatment may precipitate acute gout, and in the first three months colchicine or an anti-inflammatory drug should be prescribed as prophylaxis.

Attention to associated alcoholic liver disease and hypertension should not be neglected.

Course

Successful restoration of normal blood uric acid reduces the risk of gout and in time will lead to resorption of tophi.

Pseudogout and calcium pyrophosphate deposition disease (CPDD)

This crystal-induced arthritis is almost as frequent as gout amongst the elderly. A prerequisite is the deposition of calcium pyrophosphate in joint cartilage.

Symptoms

Like gout, pseudogout often begins at night and can be precipitated by incidental illness or surgery. Invariably, a single joint is involved and in 50% of cases this is the knee. The wrist, elbow, ankle and hip are affected less commonly and small joints are rarely involved. Acute pain and swelling may be accompanied by fever. Less commonly, chronic polyarticular pain and stiffness are associated with a picture of widespread chondrocalcinosis and osteoarthritis. Superimposed on this chronic picture may be episodes of acute inflammation.

Signs

The features of intense inflammation are seen with tenderness, erythema and swelling. As with gout, oedema may be extensive when a wrist or ankle joint is involved.

Chronic symptoms may be associated with the clinical findings of osteoarthritis, mild features of inflammation and small, persistent effusions.

Differential diagnosis

The acute attack resembles any of the disorders which may be associated with acute monoarthritis. A hot swollen knee in an elderly person is most likely to be caused by pseudogout.

Chondrocalcinosis is a common finding in the elderly and 25% of those over 70 years of age have changes in the knees. Pain due to associated osteoarthritis or incidental acute arthritis such as gout or sepsis should not be confused with pseudogout on the basis of the radiological appearance.

The disorganized joints of Charcot arthropathy may be associated with chondrocalcinosis and calcium pyrophosphate crystals may be observed in the synovial fluid.

An acute arthritis of the fingers or other joints may be due to calcific periarthritis. This is a distinct but uncommon disorder which may be familial.

Calcific tendonitis, usually of the supraspinatus tendon, may induce severe pain, florid inflammation and a joint effusion. In this and calcific periarthritis, calcium hydroxyapatite and not pyrophosphate is found near, but not in, the joint cavity.

In some patients with osteoarthritis it is possible to identify crystals of calcium hydroxyapatite. These are too small to be seen by ordinary microscopes and require electron microscopy, probe analysis or other techniques for their identification. Acute inflammation is not clinically evident in these cases and there is some doubt about the aetiological significance of the findings. It is likely that they derive from damaged bone surfaces.

Investigation

Identification of calcium pyrophosphate crystals in synovial fluid is the only way of establishing the diagnosis. Small crystals may be found in large numbers in polymorphs but they are sometimes scarce and difficult to detect. In the presence of chronic symptoms, crystals may still be seen in the synovial fluid but are less numerous and the effusion may contain only modest numbers of polymorphs, sometimes in keeping with a non-inflammatory joint disease. Radiographs of involved joints invariably show chondrocalcinosis although this may be difficult to visualize. Chondrocalcinosis of the knees affects both the menisci and articular cartilage. Generalized calcification may involve the symphysis pubis, the triangular cartilage of the wrists, the hip joints, elbows and fingers (*Figure 11.4*). Radiological features of osteoarthritis are a frequent accompaniment of chondrocalcinosis. Occasionally there may be extensive loss of cartilage and bone which is presumed to be secondary to the deposition of calcium pyrophosphate.

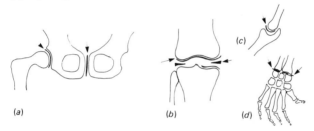

Figure 11.4   Common sites of chondrocalcinosis: (a) hip and symphysis pubis; (b) articular and meniscal cartilage of knee; (c) elbow; (d) wrist

During attacks of pseudogout, ESR and acute phase proteins are raised and there may be a leukocytosis. Unlike gout, there is no diagnostic biochemical abnormality. In young patients, or in the presence of widespread chondrocalcinosis, it is important to determine serum calcium and iron levels. Both hyperparathyroidism and haemochromatosis are associated with cartilage calcification.

Aetiology

Both calcium and pyrophosphate are widely distributed in the body but crystals of calcium pyrophosphate are only found in the joint. Subjects with chondrocalcinosis have higher levels of synovial fluid pyrophosphate and it is thought that crystal deposition is due to metabolic disturbances confined to cartilage.

Men are slightly more likely to develop chondrocalcinosis and there is a rare familial disorder of generalized chondrocalcinosis. The association between chondrocalcinosis, hyperparathyroidism and haemochromatosis may be explained by an enhancing effect of iron and calcium ions on crystal formation. However, there is no relationship between chondrocalcinosis and other causes of hypercalcaemia.

Attacks of pseudogout are precipitated by shedding of crystals from their sites of deposition. Complement activation, phagocytosis of crystals by lining cells and polymorphs and the induction of an acute phase response are involved as in acute gout.

Pathology

Calcium pyrophosphate crystals are distributed unevenly throughout the fibrocartilage of menisci, symphysis pubis and wrist as well as in hyaline cartilage. Crystals may also aggregate on the synovial lining where they may be visualized at arthroscopy.

Erosions do not occur but thinning of joint cartilage and other features of osteoarthritis are common. Whether these changes are a cause, an effect or merely incidental to chondrocalcinosis is not clear.

Treatment

Joint aspiration in the course of diagnosis helps to lessen pain. Rest and anti-inflammatory drugs such as indomethacin and naproxen will reduce inflammation over a period of days. More rapid relief can be obtained by intra-articular injection of corticosteroid. Colchicine is also effective.

There is no certain prophylactic measure and although it is important to exclude associated hyperparathyroidism, successful treatment of this disorder is often followed by progression of joint calcification. Regular anti-inflammatory drugs or colchicine may diminish the risk of recurrent acute episodes.

Course

The recurrence rate of pseudogout is highly variable. Some patients may have a single episode but others may experience two or three attacks each year.

Persistent pain is usually due to the osteoarthritis which is so often a concomitant feature.

Infective arthritis

Infectious organisms can cause arthritis either by inciting an unfavourable immune response or by invading the joint cavity. Examples of the former are reactive arthritis and rheumatic fever but these are discussed elsewhere (see Chapters 8 and 15). In some instances, both mechanisms may be involved.

Gonococcal, tuberculous, brucella, spirochaetal and viral arthritis have some specific features and are discussed separately below.

Septic or pyogenic arthritis

Symptoms

Acute pain and swelling usually affect a single joint, although several joints can be involved simultaneously. Lower limb joints are more likely to be affected and the knee is the most common site. Rigors and evidence of a preceding or concurrent infection are frequent. There may be pneumonia (as in pneumococcal arthritis) or skin infection (as in staphylococcal arthritis).

A history of chronic debilitating illness, diabetes, alcohol abuse, or preceding joint disease is usual.

Signs

The features are those described for an acute monoarthritis (*Figure 11.5*). A search for an extra-articular focus of infection may reveal signs of pneumonia, infected skin ulceration, paronychia, gall bladder disease or, rarely, bacterial endocarditis.

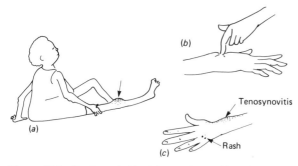

Figure 11.5 Septic arthritis: (a) a patient with quiescent rheumatoid arthritis showing inflammation of a single joint due to sepsis; (b) septic arthritis of a wrist joint producing oedema over the dorsum of the hand. A similar picture may be seen in crystal synovitis; (c) tenosynovitis of pollicis tendons with a few peripheral skin lesions in disseminated gonococcal infection

Stigmata of underlying systemic disease such as diabetes or alcoholism may be apparent. In young, apparently healthy subjects, evidence of intravenous drug abuse should be sought.

Pre-existing joint disease is most often that of RA, but other patterns of arthritis may also predispose to septic arthritis.

Differential diagnosis

Gout, pseudogout and reactive arthritis are the disorders which most closely resemble septic arthritis.

Investigation

Joint aspiration and synovial fluid analysis are the procedures of first choice. A purulent sample not containing crystals must be presumed to be infected. Gram staining and culture may isolate an organism from synovial fluid.

Liquid gas chromatographic measurement of lactic or succinic acid levels in synovial fluid has been claimed to represent a rapid discriminant test for septic arthritis.

Blood cultures give a high yield of growth because bacteraemia is an invariable feature at some stage. Culture of sputum, faeces or swabs from relevant sites may be helpful, depending on the history.

A leukocytosis is usual but is not always present. The ESR is often very high. Evidence of renal or hepatic dysfunction may be manifestations of septicaemia or predisposing disease. A macrocytic blood picture, liver enzyme changes or hyperuricaemia often denote a concealed history of alcohol abuse.

Radiographs of involved joints may be initially normal or show evidence of prior arthritis. Uncontrolled or unrecognized infection causes loss of joint space and bone erosion.

Aetiology

Septic arthritis affects men more than women and the elderly are more susceptible.

Diseases which reduce resistance to infection are commonly associated. Rheumatoid arthritis, diabetes, renal failure, alcohol abuse, lymphoma, leukaemia, immunosuppressive and corticosteroid treatment have all been incriminated. Pre-existing joint damage or prosthetic replacement also increase the risk.

Rarely, infection may be introduced during needle aspiration but usually it follows a bacteraemia. A focus of infection at another site is often identifiable.

Staphylococcus aureus is the organism involved in 70% of cases. Streptococci are the next most frequent, followed by pneumococci. *Haemophilus influenzae* has been isolated mainly from children.

Pathology

Within the joint cavity an intense inflammatory response results in accumulation of purulent fluid. A fibrinous exudate coats cartilage and synovium. Proteolytic enzymes released by polymorphs and the joint lining damage the cartilage, sometimes irreparably.

Treatment

Removal of purulent exudate by daily joint aspiration or continuous drainage is of paramount importance. The hip joint which is not accessible to needle aspiration is best drained surgically. Loculation of pus or technical problems with aspiration are further indications for surgical intervention.

Appropriate antibiotics need to be given for six weeks, initially intravenously. Intra-articular antibiotics are not required. Staphylococcal infection should be treated with two antibiotics. Symptoms can be reduced by joint splintage.

Sequential aspirates should be cultured and synovial fluid leukocytes counted in order to monitor the therapeutic response.

Weight bearing should be reintroduced gradually.

Course

Fever may take several days to remit. A joint effusion may persist for weeks but the synovial fluid neutrophil count gradually declines. Improvement may be associated with increasingly blood-stained joint aspirations. Synovial thickening, warmth, tenderness and functional impairment may be present for weeks or months after the eradication of infection.

Early aspiration and antibiotic treatment results in slow but complete recovery. Cartilage damage may lead to osteoarthritis and worsening of previous joint symptoms.

Sepsis is not a contraindication to joint replacement should this be required later. Prosthetic joints infected during insertion or immediately postoperatively are difficult to treat. Those which subsequently become infected following a bacteraemic illness often respond to conventional measures.

Gonococcal arthritis

Symptoms

This is a disease of young, healthy, sexually active subjects. There may be a history of prior urethritis but in women this may not be apparent. Symptoms sometimes coincide with menstruation or pregnancy. Rigors, fever and migratory arthralgia or arthritis may be accompanied by a rash.

Signs

During the migratory phase of the illness, transient erythema and swelling of joints may be seen. One or more of these may become persistently swollen. The rash is characteristic and comprises papules, vesicles or pustules on a grey or black base. These may be isolated or occur in crops on the extremities. Tenosynovitis is a common finding (*Figure 11.5(c)*).

Differential diagnosis

The clinical picture is readily distinguishable from other causes of septic arthritis. Very rarely, meningococcal infection can be associated with identical clinical features.

In males with a history of urethritis, distinction from reactive arthritis may be diffficult in the absence of a rash.

Investigation

As with all cases of suspected septic arthritis, joint aspiration is crucial. Migratory arthritis may be associated with small, clear effusions containing few leukocytes, and which are sterile on culture. Persistent effusions may be turbid or frankly purulent and organisms are more likely to be isolated from such aspirates.

Culture of blood, pustules, urethra, anus and oropharynx may help to identify the presence of gonococci. However, the organism is notoriously difficult to grow and special media are required.

Aetiology

The illness is caused by a bacteraemia. The presence of sterile, non-pyogenic effusions and skin lesions suggests that some features are immune-mediated. In meningococcal infection similar lesions are thought to be caused by immune complex deposition, but the evidence for this in gonococcal disease is less convincing.

In joints containing pus there is little doubt that bacteria contribute directly to the arthritis by their presence in the joint cavity.

Pathology

The skin lesions show features of a vasculitis, although organisms may also be seen on histological sections. Joints which are obviously infected exhibit the pathological features of a pyogenic arthritis.

Treatment

The standard treatment is joint immobilization, regular aspiration and intravenous penicillin for 1–2 weeks, followed by oral penicillin for two weeks. Penicillin-resistant organisms can be treated with co-trimoxazole, cefuroxime or spectinomycin.

Course

Symptoms usually remit within a week. Residual synovitis and permanent joint damage are less likely than with other types of sepsis.

Tuberculous arthritis

Tuberculosis may involve peripheral joints, tendon sheaths, sacroiliac joints or the spine.

Symptoms

Unlike pyogenic peripheral arthritis, the onset tends to be insidious, but as with other infections symptoms tend to be confined to a single joint. Involvement of a tendon sheath may cause painless swelling. The symptoms, signs and investigation of spinal infection are discussed in Chapter 6.

Signs

Peripheral joint effusion, warmth and tenderness are present but erythema and intense inflammation are absent. Fever is an occasional feature. Spinal disease may be associated with groin swelling due to tracking of pus along a psoas sheath.

Differential diagnosis

Other causes of mono-arthritis require exclusion.

Investigation

Synovial fluid may be only slightly turbid and the leukocyte count tends to be consistent with an inflammatory rather than a septic arthritis. The ESR is usually elevated but there is no leukocytosis. Staining and culture of synovial fluid identifies acid fast bacilli in only 50% of cases but synovial biopsy reveals typical granulomata in more than 90%. These often have a non-caseating appearance. Culture of synovium is also worthwhile when examination of synovial fluid has been unrewarding.

Radiographs remain normal until the disease is advanced. The Mantoux test may be strongly positive.

Aetiology

Mycobacterium tuberculosis is invariably spread from some other site which is often clinically inactive.

In Britain, Asians have a higher incidence of tuberculosis, and spinal and peripheral joint involvement are seen most frequently in this community. In the indigenous population, it is the elderly who are the most susceptible.

Pathology

Synovium becomes thickened and inflamed and granuloma formation is invariable. Cartilage and underlying bone becomes eroded over a period of many months. In the spine, infection may destroy the disc and adjacent bone. Paravertebral and psoas abscess formation is common.

Treatment

Immobilization of peripheral joints or the spine is not mandatory but splints may be of symptomatic value.

The important aspect of therapy is diagnosis and prompt institution of isoniazid, rifampicin and either streptomycin or ethambutol. These should be continued for two months and modified in the light of antibiotic sensitivities. Treatment should be continued for a further 12–18 months with isoniazid and one other preparation.

Patients can be ambulant as soon as symptoms allow. Prolonged bed rest is no longer advocated for those with spinal disease but evidence of spinal cord involvement demands surgical decompression and drainage.

Course

Occasionally joint infection may be difficult to eradicate and synovectomy may enhance chemotherapy. Vertebral bone and disc loss may be so severe that spinal fusion is necessary to eradicate pain.

Brucella arthritis

This is a rare cause of arthritis in Britain but in Spain and some other European countries it is regularly encountered.

Symptoms and signs

As with tuberculous infection, isolated peripheral joints, the spine or the sacroiliac joints may be involved. The symptoms may include night sweats and weight loss. The signs are those described for tuberculosis.

Investigation

Synovial fluid is turbid or purulent with white cell counts in the inflammatory or septic range. The organism may be grown from blood or synovial fluid. Serum agglutinins to *Brucella* can usually be detected.

A high ESR is accompanied by a normal blood leukocyte count. Mild liver dysfunction occurs in 50%.

Radiographs may show changes consistent with spinal infection, sacroiliitis or loss of peripheral joint cartilage.

Aetiology

In Britain the risk of *Brucella abortus* infection is confined to subjects who are exposed to diseased livestock. In other countries the ingestion of unpasteurized milk from goats or sheep infected with *Brucella melitensis* is the principal source of contagion.

The pathological changes are those of septic arthritis.

Treatment

Joint aspiration is important as in all septic arthritis. The need for bed rest or spinal immobilization is governed by the severity of pain. The antibiotic of choice is co-trimoxazole given for three months.

Course

As with tuberculosis, complete recovery is the rule. Spinal fusion is sometimes required.

Spirochaetal arthritis

Syphylis (Clutton's joints)

This arthritis of the knees, elbows, ankles or fingers is associated with congenital syphylis. It is of no relevance to modern clinical practice and is mentioned because finals examiners have long memories.

Lyme disease

This is a recently recognized illness in which a rash (erythema chronicum migrans) may be accompanied by fever, headache and arthritis. It affects young people and is usually transient. It was originally described in the town of Lyme, USA, but sporadic cases have been described elsewhere. It is caused by a spirochaete which is transmitted from wild animals to man by the tick *Ixodes dammini*. Tetracycline or penicillin are effective treatments.

Viral arthritis

Rubella

Arthralgia or a mild symmetrical arthritis may occur in 25% of women during or after the development of the typical rash. It is uncommon in children and men and is caused by the presence of the virus in the joints. Symptoms resolve spontaneously in a few days or weeks but a persistent synovitis lasting many months has been documented.

An identical illness may follow vaccination with the live attenuated virus. This occurs one to several weeks after injection and follows the same course as that caused by natural infection.

Hepatitis

Stiffness, arthralgia or clinical synovitis may be features of the prodrome of infectious hepatitis. The fingers are especially prone to involvement but any peripheral joint may be affected. Fever, anorexia and urticaria may be associated. The joint symptoms remit as jaundice or liver dysfunction becomes apparent.

The illness is analogous to serum sickness and is due to immune complex deposition. Hepatitis B surface antigen (HB_sAg), circulating immune complexes and a lower serum complement are common findings but HB_sAg is not always present.

Parvovirus

A symmetrical arthritis of the fingers and large joints may be associated with outbreaks of erythema infectiosum. A characteristic erythematous rash on the face and elsewhere usually accompanies the joint symptoms, although it is now recognized that arthritis may be an isolated feature.

Both children and adults may be affected. Symptoms resolve within 1–3 weeks although children may follow a more protracted course.

Arboviruses

Fever, rash and arthritis may be features of mosquito transmitted group A arboviruses. The most well known is that of Ross River virus infection which has caused epidemic outbreaks in Australia.

Other viruses

There have been infrequent descriptions of arthralgia or arthritis accompanying infection with Epstein Barr virus (with and without typical features of infectious mononucleosis), mumps, varicella, Coxsackie B and variola viruses.

Further reading

FAM, A. *et al.* (1981). Clinical and radiological aspects of pseudogout: a study of 50 cases and a review. *Can. Med. Ass. J.*, **124,** 545

FOX, I. (1981). Metabolic basis for disorders of purine nucleotide degradation. *Metabolism,* **30,** 616

GOLDENBERG, D. (1983). Postinfectious arthritis. New look at an old concept with particular attention to disseminated gonococcal infection. *Am. J. Med.*, **74,** 925

PLATT, P. (1983). Examination of synovial fluid. *Clin. Rheum. Dis.*, **9,** 51

ROSENTHAL, J. *et al.* (1980). Acute non-gonococcal infectious arthritis – evaluation of risk factors, therapy and outcome. *Arthritis Rheum.*, **23,** 889

SCOTT, J. T. (1980). Long term management of gout and hyperuricaemia. *Br. Med. J.*, **281,** 1164

12
Connective tissue diseases

The term connective tissue disease is probably the best available to describe a number of relatively uncommon disorders which share clinical and serological features. Its use is not intended to invoke any specific aetiological or pathological process although the cells and extracellular protein of connective tissue are inevitably affected by the diseases to be discussed. It may be argued that connective tissue involvement is not exclusive to these conditions. In conceding this, it may be stated that the term is now used more frequently than any of the alternative and equally inappropriate expressions such as collagen vascular and auto-immune disease.

The title encompasses the disorders of systemic lupus erythematosus (SLE), scleroderma, polymyositis and mixed connective tissue disease (MCTD). This exclusive list is somewhat arbitrary and other authors might have included Sjögren's syndrome, polyarteritis nodosa and, more pedantically, rheumatoid arthritis.

Systemic lupus erythematosus (SLE)

This connective tissue disease has a wide spectrum of clinical manifestations and severity. Involvement of kidneys and other internal organs is frequent. It is a disease which mainly affects young women.

131

Symptoms

The disease may begin suddenly with fever, arthritis, rash or other major manifestations. It is just as likely to evolve over many months or even years with periodic bouts of ill health affecting different systems. Fatigue and weight loss are common but non-specific complaints.

Arthralgia or painful swelling of joints is the most common feature and is seen in more than 90% of patients. Fingers, wrists and knees are the most commonly affected. Stiffness occurs but neither this nor pain cause the degree of physical disability seen in RA. Muscle weakness may be prominent.

Skin manifestations occur in 75%. A history of Raynaud's phenomenon, photosensitivity rashes, urticaria, other less specific rashes and thinning of the hair may be elicited.

A history of chest pain, often pleuritic in nature, may be recalled. Such episodes may be associated with dyspnoea and wrongly attributed to lung infection. Abdominal pain is less frequent.

Depression, headaches, convulsions, confusional states or psychotic behaviour may all be relevant. Neurological symptoms may be an early manifestation and when they occur as isolated events the diagnosis may be exceptionally difficult.

Mouth, nose or pharyngeal ulceration can cause great discomfort. Bleeding and discharge from these sites may occur.

Peripheral oedema may be the first indication of renal involvement. Severe renal failure may cause fatigue, nausea, pruritus, convulsions and confusion.

Symptoms worsen after exposure to ultraviolet light and during menstruation, pregnancy or infections. The ingestion of several different drugs including oestrogen oral contraceptives can also induce flares of the disease.

Signs

In severe, active disease, patients may be febrile, pale and look unwell. Others have mild disease with little constitutional disturbance. Examination of potential sites of involvement may reveal the features listed below.

Skin

The classical butterfly rash over the cheeks and nose occurs in less than 50%. It is an erythematous eruption, often induced or accentuated by exposure to sunlight (*Figure 12.1*). Photosensitivity may be manifest by rashes of other exposed areas. These may be erythematous, macular, papular, urticarial or bullous. Patchy alopecia is common but is sometimes concealed or dismissed by patients. Scarring alopecia may be associated with discoid lupus, a distinctive and circumscribed rash which most often occurs as an independent disorder. It usually affects the face and may be associated with telangiectasia, depigmentation and scarring.

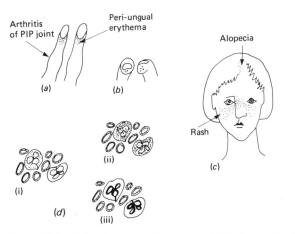

Figure 12.1 Systemic lupus erythematosus. (a) Peri-ungual erythema and arthritis of the PIP joints; (b) finger tip infarcts; (c) butterfly rash and alopecia; (d) three patterns of glomerulonephritis as seen by light microscopy: (i) focal proliferative; (ii) diffuse proliferative; (iii) membranous

Raynaud's phenomenon may be suggested by cool, cyanosed digits. There may be erythema of the palms, finger tips and around the nails (*Figure 12.1(a)*). Nail fold and finger tip infarcts may be associated with characteristic brown flecks adjacent to the nails or scarring of the finger tips (*Figure 12.1(b)*).

Purpura of the feet may be a feature of cutaneous vasculitis. At pressure sites it may denote the presence of thrombocytopenia. Livedo reticularis is a blotchy discolouration of the extremities, sometimes seen in health and commonly in SLE. Scattered, painful nodules or panniculitis are the least common cutaneous manifestations (lupus profundus).

Joints

Joint pain may be seen without signs of inflammation but intermittent swelling of the finger joints, wrists and other sites often occurs. Deformities and subluxation are rare and when they arise are often reversible. They are due to tendon inflammation and do not imply a destructive arthritis.

Muscles

Disuse wasting may occur in association with arthritis. A proximal myopathy with wasting and weakness may be due to a true myositis. Myopathy may also be secondary to corticosteroid treatment.

Chest

A history of pleuritic chest pain may indicate pleurisy or pericarditis. Pleural and pericardial friction rubs may be audible even in the absence of a suggestive history. There may be signs of a pleural effusion and occasionally crackles at the lung bases.

Mouth and nose

Ulceration is often severe and associated with other major manifestations. Secondary infection and moniliasis may complicate mucosal ulceration. Difficulty in eating may contribute to the debility and misery of severe disease activity.

Abdomen

Slight enlargement of liver or spleen is found in 25% of patients at some time. Abdominal tenderness is an occasional finding.

Lymph nodes

Generalized lymphadenopathy is a common finding but has no special significance.

Nervous system

Neurological features are protean. Psychiatric illness may be manifest as depression, confusional states or psychotic behaviour. Grand mal, focal and temporal lobe epilepsy is common. Headaches may be benign or associated with meningism. Cerebellar signs, hemiplegia, paraplegia and peripheral neuropathy have all been documented. Retinal exudates or papilloedema occasionally occur.

Kidneys

Hypertension or the oedema of nephrotic syndrome may be the only outward evidence of renal disease.

Differential diagnosis

An illness of young women affecting joints and other systems either simultaneously or sequentially is highly suggestive of SLE. Classical features such as a butterfly rash increase this likelihood but the ultimate diagnosis depends on compatible laboratory findings.

The arthritis can be distinguished from RA by its non-deforming nature and the lack of erosions on radiographs. Rheumatoid factors occur in 10% of patients with SLE and a positive antinuclear factor (ANF) test occurs in a similar proportion of RA patients but antibodies against double stranded DNA are rare in RA.

Raynaud's phenomenon, arthritis, pleurisy, pericarditis and myositis are also consistent with scleroderma and mixed connective tissue disease. In the absence of other clinical features, diagnosis may be dependent on the interpretation of laboratory tests but even then it may be difficult and somewhat arbitrary.

Involvement of one or a few anatomical sites without a typical history of multisystem disease often requires exclusion of a wide range of disorders. A proportion of patients with idiopathic thrombocytopenia purpura subsequently develop other features of SLE.

One major difficulty commonly encountered is the distinction of incidental disease from active SLE. Sepsis is a common complication and like SLE may cause fever. Rising titres of anti-double stranded DNA, and reduced serum complement levels are consistent with active SLE whereas an increasing C reactive protein (CRP) would suggest infection. Pneumonia, infective meningitis and septicaemia are difficult to exclude in the very ill patients. Psychosis or confusion due to uraemia, fever, steroid treatment or electrolyte imbalance is sometimes impossible to distinguish from SLE involvement of the nervous system.

Investigation

In suspected cases, laboratory investigations are crucial to the diagnosis.

Haematology

A mild hypochromic or normochromic anaemia is common. Haemolysis occurs in less than 10% at some time but a positive Coombs test is seen in 25%. Lymphopenia is usual in active SLE. Neutropenia occurs in 50% and thrombocytopenia in 25%. A circulating anticoagulant (lupus anticoagulant) occurs in 5% and causes prolongation of the partial thromboplastin time. Paradoxically, it increases susceptibility to venous and arterial thrombosis and does not cause bleeding.

Routine biochemistry

Increased blood urea and creatinine imply severe renal involvement.

Minor liver dysfunction is common. Salicylates ingested by SLE patients often cause a rise of liver enzymes. Heart failure, hepatotoxic drugs and SLE itself may be associated with similar changes. The severe liver derangement of chronic active hepatitis may be associated with extrahepatic clinical features which resemble SLE but this is a distinct and separate disorder.

Myositis and haemolysis are also causes of increased serum aspartate transferase (AST).

Serology

Nearly all patients with SLE have positive tests for ANF. Detection of high titre of antibodies against double stranded DNA (*see* Chapter 3) is almost specific for SLE. Titres of both ANF and double stranded DNA (dsDNA) antibody may fluctuate with disease activity.

Rarely, patients with clinical SLE have a negative ANF test. Such patients may have anti-Ro antibodies (also known as anti-SSA). Others with a positive ANF test but no antibodies against dsDNA may have anti-Sm antibodies. Negative ANF and anti-Ro test make a diagnosis of SLE unlikely. Antibodies against two other soluble antigens are often present. These are anti-RNP and anti-La (also called anti-SSB). Anti-RNP occurs in 40% and is often associated with anti-Sm. Anti-La antibodies occur in 15% and are nearly always seen in association with anti-Ro. Those with anti-Ro and La tend not to exhibit antibodies against RNP and Sm. Total serum haemolytic complement (CH_{50}), C3 or C4 may be reduced in active SLE.

Anti-cardiolipin antibodies give rise to a biological false positive test for syphylis in which the VDRL is positive but specific tests for treponemal infection are negative. The lupus anticoagulant is often associated with this finding.

Kidneys

In addition to blood urea and creatinine it is useful to estimate creatinine clearance or some other measure of GFR. Urine should always be examined for cells, casts, protein and blood. The presence of protein should be quantified. Most patients with SLE have immunoglobulins in their glomeruli but kidney biopsy is justifiable only when there are urinary abnormalities or a reduced GFR.

Chest

A chest radiograph may reveal a pleural effusion, aspiration of which usually yields fluid with a high protein content. Occasionally there may be streaky basal shadowing and progressive diminution of lung volume (shrinking lung) in which respiratory function tests reveal a restrictive defect. This feature is thought to be caused by stiffening of the diaphragm.

Suspected pericarditis can be investigated by ECG and echocardiography. Occasionally, echocardiograms reveal small valve vegetations (Libman Sacks endocarditis) but these are of no consequence.

Congenital heartblock has been documented amongst the offspring of mothers with SLE. This complication is associated with the transmission of anti-Ro antibodies.

Skin

Biopsy of involved and uninvolved sites may show evidence of immunoglobulin and complement deposition at the dermal-epidermal junction (lupus band test). This is neither apparent in all cases nor specific for SLE.

Nervous system

Both affective and organic psychiatric problems may arise and their discrimination is difficult.

The demonstration of cells or increased protein in CSF and abnormal EEG or brain scans favour organic disease but these cannot differentiate between neurological symptoms caused by SLE, uraemia, hypertension or infection. Brain scans using radiolabelled oxygen have been claimed to represent a more sensitive index of CNS involvement but this test is not widely available and the claims are unsubstantiated. CT scans of the brain are often abnormal but lack of specificity detracts from their discriminatory value. Nuclear magnetic resonance (NMR) may be more sensitive but equally lacking in specificity.

Aetiology

The disease is nine times more frequent in women than men. It is more common in North America than in Europe. Negroes, Malays and Chinese are more susceptible than Caucasians. There is a weak positive association with HLA DR2 and DR3 and a negative association with HLA DR4 and DR5.

Patients with hereditary complement deficiency often have SLE. The frequency of this association varies from 20–50%, dependent on the pattern of complement disorder. Hereditary C2 deficiency is the most common but insufficiency of C4, C1q, C5, C8 or other complement components has been described.

In general, SLE patients appear to have reduced numbers of C3b receptors on their erythrocytes. It is not clear how this may be related to the aetiology, but complement assists in the disposal of immune complexes by C3 opsonization and C3 disruption of antigen–antibody lattices. A defective complement system may thus hinder solubilization and removal of immune complexes.

A wide range of functional lymphocyte abnormalities has been described. In the circulation. cytotoxic-suppressor T cells are reduced, spontaneous cytotoxicity by natural killer (NK) cells is diminished and interleukin-1 production and its effect on T cells is defective. It is uncertain how these phenomena are related to the vigorous B cell synthesis of antibodies which characterizes the disease.

Immune complexes of anti-dsDNA–DNA and anti-ssDNA–DNA are found in the circulation and at involved tissue sites, especially in the skin and kidneys. Activation of complement by complexes is presumed to initiate an injurious inflammatory response. Anti-DNA antibodies belong to both IgG and IgM classes and show a spectrum of avidity for antigen. High avidity antibodies may be associated with renal disease.

The antibodies against Sm, RNP and other extractable antigens do not exert any proven effect through immune complexes. A panoply of additional antibodies such as lymphocytotoxic and anti-neuronal antibodies play an equally uncertain role.

Some drugs can induce reversible SLE. Neurological and renal disease do not occur but most other features have been described. Hydralazine and procainamide show some structural similarity and both may cause SLE, especially in patients who are slow acetylators. The total dose of drug and the presence of HLA DR4 increase the risk. Women receiving hydralazine and who are both slow acetylators and HLA DR4 positive are almost certain to develop symptoms. Isoniazid, D-penicillamine, phenytoin and practolol have also been incriminated. Both hydralazine and isoniazid inhibit C4 binding and may interrupt its role in the removal of immune complexes. Antibodies to histones are common but anti-dsDNA and anti-SM are rare in drug-induced disease.

Pathology

Joints

Synovial tissue is hyperplastic with non-specific sub-synovial inflammation. Fibrinoid necrosis of synovial vessels has been described. Synovial fluid tends to be non-inflammatory in nature.

Skin

Varying degrees of keratosis, epidermal atrophy and chronic inflammation around vessels and the dermal–epidermal junction occur where immunoglobulins and complement may also be detected.

Kidneys

Immunoglobulin or complement can be detected in the glomeruli of nearly all patients with SLE. Clinical renal disease is associated with three major histopathological patterns of nephritis:

1. Focal proliferative – in which cellular proliferation affects some but not all glomeruli. This is associated with mild renal disease.
2. Diffuse proliferative – associated with dense proliferation of all or most glomeruli. Patients with this picture have more urine abnormalities, greater impairment of GFR and are less responsive to treatment. Nephrotic syndrome is an occasional feature.
3. Membranous – thickened glomerular basement membranes are associated with the nephrotic syndrome (see Figure 12.1(d)).

These patterns are not always constant with time nor can they be confidently predicted on the basis of the clinical findings.

Nervous system

Despite a striking array of neurological features, pathological changes in the brain are sparse and non-specific. Vasculitis is not seen.

Treatment

Not all patients with SLE have a life-threatening disease and treatment should be designed to lessen rather than increase the hazards. Those with arthritis, skin disease and minimal internal organ disease may be managed with anti-inflammatory drugs, analgesics and antimalarials. Exposure to strong sunlight and sun lamps should be avoided and the skin protected in sunny weather.

Small or modest doses of corticosteroids are necessary for pleurisy, pericarditis, lung involvement, thrombocytopenia, myositis and haemolysis. Nervous system manifestations may respond to modest doses (30–60 mg) of prednisolone. Larger doses and immunosuppressive drugs have no proven value. Anticonvulsants are used when necessary. Severe or progressive renal disease may be contained by prednisolone. Concomitant immunosuppressive agents are conventionally prescribed and may exert a beneficial effect. Azathioprine is the safest but cyclophosphamide is also used. Rapidly progressive renal disease with diffuse proliferative and crescentic changes on biopsy may be treated with pulses of intravenous methyl prednisolone (1.0 g daily for four days). Immunosuppressive agents and plasmapheresis may be added to this regime. Hypertension should be vigorously treated. Hydralazine is not precluded from use despite its ability to induce an SLE illness. Long-term corticosteroid treatment should be maintained at the smallest dose compatible with relief of symptoms. Alternate day therapy may be adequate. End-stage kidney disease may be successfully managed by dialysis or renal transplantation.

Course

Five year survival exceeds 90% and has improved in the last decade. This may be due to the recognition of milder disease and more circumspect use of harmful treatments.

Nervous system involvement and diffuse proliferative nephritis have the worst prognosis. Pregnancy may worsen the disease and the risk of spontaneous abortion is increased. Infection is a major cause of mortality. This is partly due to the disease and partly to the effects of treatment on the immune system. Corticosteroid treatment is associated with a long catalogue of side effects including avascular necrosis, a complication seen regularly in SLE. An increased death rate from intracerebral and cardiovascular disease has been attributed to acceleration of atheroma by corticosteroids.

Scleroderma

This is a rare multisystem disease which affects women more than men and is characterized by fibrosis of skin and other organs.

Symptoms

Raynaud's phenomenon is a constant feature and may precede other symptoms by years. Stiffness and tightening of the skin over the fingers may impede function and the finger tips may be intermittently painful or associated with small ulcers. Patients often fail to emphasize involvement of facial skin, which is obvious to even a casual observer. Swelling of the feet, ankles and fingers is often an early complaint. Pain and stiffness of peripheral joints and proximal muscles may occur.

Internal organ disease may develop early or late. Heartburn, indigestion and dysphagia suggest oesophageal involvement. Diarrhoea, bloating, constipation and weight loss imply disease of the small or large bowel. Chest pain may have the features of pleurisy or pericarditis and exertional dyspnoea is a further indication of lung or heart involvement.

Signs

In the early stages of disease there may be puffy swelling of the digits, feet and face without obvious skin tightening. The fingers may later become fixed in flexion due to skin and tendon contraction, smooth and shiny due to skin tightening (sclerodacty-ly), or cool and cyanosed due to Raynaud's phenomenon (*Figure 12.2*). The skin over the dorsum of the hands may be difficult to pinch and over the extremities and trunk may appear thickened and immobile. There may be ulcers or scars on the fingertips. The face develops a characteristic thin appearance with loss of forehead wrinkles, a reduced oral aperture and taut shiny skin over the nose.

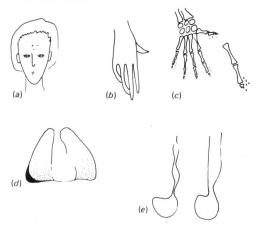

Figure 12.2 Scleroderma. (a) Loss of facial wrinkles, thin face, pinched nose, telangiectasia and reduced oral aperature; (b) sclerodactyly with smooth taut skin; (c) terminal tuft erosions and subcutaneous calcification; (d) pleural effusion and fibrosing alveolitis; (e) barium swallow showing normal peristalsis on the left and an atonic, dilated oesophagus on the right

Telangiectasia over the face, lips or trunk are common. The constellation of radiological calcinosis (C), Raynaud's phenomenon (R), sclerodacytyly (S) and telangiectasia (T) is often referred to as the CRST syndrome. These features may be associated with oesophageal involvement (CREST) syndrome – 'E' representing oesophagus.

Joint tenderness is common and intermittent swelling of finger joints may occur. Tendons become thickened and their movement may be associated with palpable crepitus.

Proximal muscle wasting is often due to disuse. As in SLE, weakness, wasting and pain may be due to a myositis. Apart from occasional sensory impairment in the distribution of one or more divisions of the fifth cranial nerve, neurological signs are not a feature.

Pericardial and pleural rubs, signs of pleural effusions and crackles at the lung bases are signs of cardiac or pulmonary involvement. An irregular pulse and other features of heart failure may be evidence of myocardial fibrosis and cor pulmonale may complicate lung disese. Hypertension can be severe and associated with a rapid decline of renal function. Abdominal distension and emaciation are signs of small bowel disease and malabsorption. Faecal loading of the caecum and colon indicate large bowel involvement. Stigmata of liver disease may suggest the presence of primary biliary cirrhosis, which is an occasional association.

Differential diagnosis

Raynaud's phenomenon is always a prominent feature of scleroderma but is also seen in SLE, mixed connective tissue disease and as an isolated disorder (Raynaud's disease).

The early skin changes may resemble myxoedema. They should not be confused with localized scleroderma (morphoea). This is a confined, plaque-like rash, sometimes distributed in a linear fashion on the face, limbs or trunk. It is often associated with atrophy of underlying muscle and bone. Sclerederma is a rare puffiness of the skin which has a superficial resemblance to scleroderma. Eosinophilic fasciitis is also rare but resembles scleroderma more closely. Eosinophils in the blood and subcutaneous tissue are associated with fibrosis of fascia, induration of skin and restricted elbow and shoulder movement. The onset is often acute and neither Raynaud's phenomenon nor internal organ involvement are seen. Some of these patients develop serious blood dyscrasias. Occasionally, the arthritis of scleroderma may be florid and suggestive of RA. Myositis in early disease may be difficult to distinguish from polymyositis.

Investigations

Non-specific haematological evidence of chronic inflammation may include mild anaemia and an elevated ESR. Routine biochemistry is often normal. An elevated serum aspartate transferase (AST) in the presence of a normal alkaline phosphatase usually indicates myositis. A rising urea and creatinine are portents of rapidly progressive disease.

Skin biopsy is sometimes warranted but tends to show non-specific changes until the disease is well established and clinically obvious. Exclusion of eosinophilic fasciitis requires a deep biopsy.

Radiographs of the hands may reveal calcinosis and terminal tuft resorption (*see Figure 12.2(c)*). Occasionally, joint erosions are present.

Myositis may be demonstrated by an increased serum CPK, EMG and muscle biopsy.

Evidence of oesophageal involvement can be detected by manometry which shows loss of normal peristalsis. Barium swallow is less sensitive but in late disease may show disordered peristalsis or a distended, akinetic oesophagus (*see Figure 12.2(e)*). Small bowel barium studies may reveal duodenal or ileal dilatation with flocculation. A plain abdominal film demonstrating distended bowel or gross constipation reflects large bowel involvement. This can be confirmed by barium enema. Evidence of malabsorption may be suggested by pronounced anaemia or macrocytosis. Faecal fat collection and xylose tolerance are confirmatory investigations.

Chest radiographs may reveal pleural effusion or thickening and not infrequently increased shadowing of the lung bases (*see Figure 12.2(d)*). In advanced pulmonary disease there may be extensive fibrotic changes. Respiratory function tests often reveal defects of restriction and diffusion despite normal radiographs.

Radiographic evidence of an enlarged heart may be due to heart failure, pericardial effusion or myocardial fibrosis. An ECG commonly reveals conduction abnormalities such as varying degrees of heart block. Echocardiography may confirm a pericardial effusion.

A positive ANF test occurs in 90%, sometimes with a nucleolar pattern of staining. Anti-dsDNA antibodies are not seen. In 30% of patients antibodies against a nuclear antigen in the centromere region can be detected. This anticentromere antibody (ACA) is associated with the CRST syndrome. An antibody against another extractable antigen called Scl-70 occurs in 20%. It is unusual to demonstrate both Scl-70 and ACA in the same patient. IgM RF occurs in 10%.

Aetiology

The disease occurs in all racial groups. Women are affected five times more frequently than men and there is a weak association with HLA DR5.

An illness resembling scleroderma has been described following exposure to industrial vinyl chloride. Susceptibility to this disorder is slightly increased by possession of HLA DR5 and more severe disease by HLA DR3. The ingestion of adulterated rapeseed oil in Spain has caused a scleroderma-like illness in some patients with the toxic epidemic syndrome. Raynaud's phenomenon, cutaneous fibrosis and lung involvement may occur. There may be a relationship between this syndrome and HLA DR3 and DR4.

Patients who develop graft versus host disease may also have a clinical picture resembling scleroderma. Unmistakable and rapidly progressive scleroderma has been described in association with malignant disease. Industrial exposure to silica dust may be an aetiological factor. Silicone mammoplasty has been associated with a scleroderma-like disease.

An immunological response is manifest by the range of antibodies already discussed. Antibodies to Types 1 and 4 collagen may also occur, the latter showing some association with lung involvement. Immune complexes can be demonstrated in 30%. Several abnormalities of lymphocyte function have been described but these are not impressive and await further study. Attempts to link the genetic, immunological and environmental factors discussed above with the pathology described below have been difficult. The fibroblasts in scleroderma produce excessive collagen. It has been suggested that they are either stimulated by a circulating lymphokine or represent an overactive clone which has displaced normal fibroblasts.

Pathology

Early in the disease, inflammatory changes in skin, synovium and tendons may be associated with immunoglobulin deposition. As the disease progresses, intense fibrosis develops. A similar fibrotic process affects myocardium, lungs and the gastrointestinal tract.

Dense collagen replaces the muscle of the oesophagus and other involved areas of the gut.

Intimal hyperplasia of small arteries of the fingers, lungs and kidneys accounts for some of the more serious clinical sequelae. In the microcirculation, capillaries are diminished in number and display a characteristic tortuosity and dilatation.

Treatment

There is no really effective treatment for progressive scleroderma. D-penicillamine and colchicine may retard the disease but their effects are unpredictable. Corticosteroids have a limited role in the management of painful serositis unresponsive to other anti-inflammatory agents. Plasmapheresis and immunosuppressive drugs have been claimed to offer benefits. Many other treatments have been advocated without good evidence of efficacy.

Aggressive treatment of hypertension with vasodilators such as prazosin and captopril may avert renal failure. Uncontrollable hypertension and end-stage kidney disease can be managed by nephrectomy and dialysis.

The treatment of Raynaud's phenomenon is warm clothing and gloves. Nifedipine and the serotinin receptor blocker, ketanserin, are worth trying.

Course

The outcome of scleroderma is highly variable. Some have a rapidly progressive illness spanning months. The majority have a disease which worsens slowly or sporadically over many years.

The CRST syndrome sometimes follows a benign course but its presence does not exclude the development of serious internal organ disease.

Polymyositis and dermatomyositis

This disorder of muscle is similar to the myositis of SLE, scleroderma and mixed connective tissue disease. When accompanied by a rash it is called dermatomyositis.

Symptoms

Weakness is a prominent complaint. Proximal muscle stiffness and pain are variable features. Patients experience difficulty in dressing, combing their hair and climbing stairs. The onset tends to be insidious but may be sudden. A history of arthralgia and Raynaud's phenomenon occurs in 30%. Swelling of the fingers may be an early and transient symptom. In severe disease, dysphagia, dysphonia and dyspnoea may be encountered. Weight loss, change of bowel habit, haemoptysis or rectal bleeding may suggest the presence of an associated neoplasm.

Signs

Proximal muscle weakness can be demonstrated by asking patients to lift head or legs against resistance while lying supine. Muscle tenderness occurs in less than 50% and wasting develops in patients with severe progressive disease.

A pink, erythematous rash occurring over the extensor surfaces of the finger joints is characteristic of dermatomyositis. Similar discolouration may occur over the elbows, forearms, knees and thighs. Peri-orbital oedema and erythema (so-called heliotrope discolouration) is an occasional accompaniment (*Figure 12.3(a)* and *(b)*).

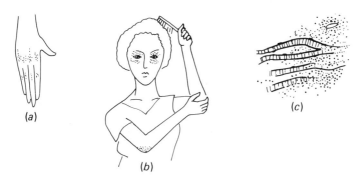

Figure 12.3   Dermatomyositis and polymyositis. (a) Rash over dorsum of fingers in dermatomyositis; (b) rash on eyelids (heliotrope discolouration) and elbows. The patient is unable to brush her hair with one arm because of proximal muscle weakness; (c) histology of involved striated muscle showing necrosis of muscle fibres and infiltration with chronic inflammatory cells

Swallowing difficulties are due to involvement of pharyngeal or oesophageal muscles. Dyspnoea usually reflects respiratory muscle disease but may occasionally be associated with signs of fibrosing alveolitis or infection. Finger clubbing, pleural effusions or abdominal signs usually indicate underlying malignancy. Cardiac arrhythmias are evidence of myocardial involvement but this is a rare manifestation.

A distinctive pattern of dermatomyositis is seen in children (*see* Chapter 15).

Differential diagnosis

Proximal myopathy may be caused by muscular dystrophy, hypothyroidism, thyrotoxicosis, diabetes, steroids and disturbed calcium or potassium metabolism. Muscle wasting and weakness occur in the cachexia of malignancy and severe malnutrition. Myositis associated with other connective tissue diseases should be suggested by the presence of other clinical features. Polymyalgia rheumatica is distinguished by a history of pain, stiffness and tenderness with little weakness.

Investigations

Elevation of ESR is usual. In active disease the serum enzymes CPK and AST are elevated. Muscle enzymes are also raised in muscular dystrophy and hypothyroidism. Myoglobinuria may be detected when muscle necrosis is pronounced (rhabdomyolysis).

Electromyography (EMG) is invariably abnormal and may show characteristic alterations of electric potentials. Diagnosis is best established by muscle biopsy taken from a site not subjected to EMG, the needle of which may evoke local inflammation.

Antinuclear antibodies occur in 20% but antibodies against dsDNA are not seen. Antibodies against the extractable nuclear antigen Jo-1 are associated with pulmonary involvement.

A chest radiograph may show increased basal shadowing due to fibrosing alveolitis. Pulmonary opacities due to aspiration pneumonia may follow pharyngeal involvement. Manometry or a barium swallow may reveal abnormal motility of the lower part of the oesophagus similar to that of scleroderma.

Respiratory function tests may help to monitor chest muscle involvement and fibrosing alveolitis. Electrocardiographs may show conduction defects when the myocardium is affected.

In 10% of patients with polymyositis–dermatomyositis there is an associated malignancy. Beyond a chest radiograph and careful examination of the breasts it is rarely rewarding to search energetically for an occult tumour.

Aetiology

Women are affected twice as frequently as men and unlike some closely related disorders the onset tends to be in middle age or later.

A myositis may follow influenza and *Toxoplasma* infections and it is therefore possible that some patients with polymyositis have an infectious illness. Electron microscopy has revealed inclusions which may be viral, but these are not a consistent finding.

The association of myositis with several connective tissue diseases suggests an immunological disorder. Lymphocytes from patients with polymyositis exhibit *in vitro* cytotoxicity against skeletal muscle but apart from the association with anti-Jo-1 antibodies other evidence that this is an immune disorder is lacking.

The link with malignant disease is stronger for dermatomyositis than muscle disease alone but the mechanism of association is unknown.

Pathology

Involved muscle is characterized by fibre atrophy and inflammatory cell infiltration, principally by lymphocytes (see Figure 12.3(c)). The intensity of the cellular infiltrate lessens with time and clinical improvement. Muscle regeneration and necrosis may occur simultaneously.

Skin changes are those of atrophy, perivasculitis and deposition of mucin, a finding considered by some to be highly characteristic.

Immunoglobulin and complement can be found in muscle. The significance of this is uncertain because similar observations have been made in degenerative muscle diseases.

Treatment

Corticosteroids usually have a beneficial effect on symptoms, paralleled by improvement of laboratory indices. Initial doses of prednisolone may need to be high (40–60 mg) and if the response is limited or if high doses are required for long periods, the addition of azathioprine or another immunosuppressive agent is desirable. Methotrexate has been used with success.

Physiotherapy can help patients to improve the power of recovering of residual healthy muscle fibres.

Treatment of an associated neoplasm may induce remission of the polymyositis.

Course

Some patients present with a life-threatening illness in which respiratory embarrassment may be complicated by chest infection. Their response to corticosteroids is usually no less gratifying than those with a more insidious presentation.

Treatment may be required for many years or even indefinitely. Apparent remission may be followed by relapse. Muscle weakness caused by corticosteroids may be difficult to differentiate from that of the disease under treatment.

The five-year mortality rate is 30%. Patients with malignant disease obviously have a worse outlook.

Mixed connective tissue disease (MCTD)

This is a controversial diagnosis because some believe that it represents an entity whereas others argue that the clinical and laboratory features can be encompassed by the spectrum of SLE, scleroderma and polymyositis.

Historical

A series of patients with overlapping features of SLE and scleroderma, no renal disease and a benign course was associated with speckled staining for ANF and antibodies against an extractable nuclear antigen (ENA). Subsequently, the speckled staining pattern and ENA were shown to be due to several ENAs (*see* Chapter 3). One of these, anti-RNP, was thought to have a strong association with the clinical picture originally described.

It is now recognized that some of those patients initially categorized as MCTD later developed scleroderma or SLE and their course was not always benign. Antibodies against RNP occur in SLE and other connective tissue diseases and the specificity of this antibody for MCTD is no longer accepted.

Despite these reservations there remains a group of patients who have neither classical SLE nor scleroderma. They may have high titres of anti-RNP and lack anti-dsDNA. The diagnosis of MCTD is thus one of convenience for patients whose illness cannot be confidently attributed to a major connective tissue disease. Whether or not they have a distinct disease may be argued for many years to come.

Clinical

Raynaud's phenomenon, swollen fingers, arthritis, pulmonary fibrosis and myositis have been the most consistent features described. The arthritis sometimes dominates the picture.

The development of neurological, renal or gastrointestinal involvement makes the diagnosis unlikely.

Investigation

An elevated ESR and mild leukopenia may be seen. The antinuclear factor test is positive but antibodies against dsDNA and Sm antigen are absent. High titres of antibody against RNP are a mandatory diagnostic feature.

Radiographs of the hands may reveal calcinosis with joint subluxation and erosions. Views of the chest may show fibrosing alveolitis or pleural effusion.

Muscle involvement may be confirmed by the investigations described in the section on polymyositis (p. 150).

Treatment

Symptomatic treatment with non-steroidal anti-inflammatory drugs is often adequate. Corticosteroids may be required for myositis or lung involvement.

Course

The prognosis is much better than that of SLE, scleroderma and polymyositis. However, it must be remembered that MCTD is by definition a diagnosis which excludes serious internal organ disease.

Further reading

AUSTIN, H. *et al.* (1983). Prognosic factors in lupus nephritis. Contribution of renal histologic data. *Am. J. Med.,* **75,** 382

BOHAN, A. and PETER, J. (1975). Polymyositis and dermatomyositis. *N. Engl. J. Med.,* **292,** 344

BOTSTEIN, G. *et al.* (1982). Fibroblast selection in scleroderma. An alternative model of fibrosis. *Arthritis Rheum.,* **25,** 189

BUNCH, T. (1981). Prednisone and azathioprine for polymyositis – a long term follow up. *Arthritis Rheum.,* **24,** 45

DINANT, H. *et al.* (1982). Alternative modes of cyclophosphamide and azathioprine therapy in lupus nephritis. *Ann. Intern. Med.,* **96,** 723

FRITZLER, M. *et al.* (1980). The Crest syndrome – a distinct serologic entity with anticentromere antibodies. *Am. J. Med.,* **69,** 520

SNAITH, M. (1983). Classifying lupus. *Br. Med. J.,* **287,** 377

STEEN, V. *et al.* (1985). Pulmonary involvement in systemic sclerosis (scleroderma). *Arthritis Rheum.,* **28,** 759

WILLIAMSON, G. *et al.* (1983). Clinical characteristics of patients with rheumatic disorders who possess antibodies against RNP particles. *Arthritis Rheum.,* **26,** 509

13
Polyarteritis nodosa (PAN)

This is a rare disorder with a distinctive clinical pattern. It has little resemblance to other diseases in which arteritis is a feature. Unlike the connective tissue diseases, men are affected more than women.

Symptoms

The onset is usually sudden and accompanied by malaise, fever and weight loss. Arthralgia, muscle pain, rashes, paraesthesiae, weakness and abdominal pain are amongst the most frequent initial complaints. Gastrointestinal bleeding may complicate abdominal pain and testicular involvement may cause a distressing orchitis. Blurring of vision sometimes indicates retinal vasculitis; confusional states and stroke syndromes imply involvement of intracranial vessels. Dyspnoea and wheezing are occasional symptoms.

Signs

Dense purpura, mainly of the extremities but also of the trunk and mucosal surfaces, is common (*Figure 13.1(a)*). Digital infarcts and gangrene may occur. Urticaria and livedo reticularis have also been described.

Joint pain may be accompanied by transient swelling but persistent synovitis is not seen.

Clinical signs of peripheral neuropathy or mononeuritis multiplex occur in 60%. Retinal vasculitis is manifest by retinal haemorrhages and exudates. These need to be distinguished from hypertensive retinopathy. Evidence of central nervous system involvement may include confusion, hemiplegia, cranial nerve palsies or transient ischaemic attacks.

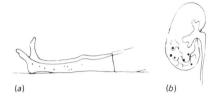

(a)   (b)

Figure 13.1 Polyarteritis nodosa. (a) Left foot drop due to mononeuritis affecting the common peroneal nerve and rash on the legs due to cutaneous vasculitis; (b) renal arteriogram showing small aneurysms in the lower pole of the kidney

Abdominal symptoms are often accompanied by signs of an acute abdomen with tenderness, guarding and loss of bowel sounds.

Examination of the chest may reveal wheezing or crackles.

Hypertension occurs in 50% and may be associated with rapid deterioration of kidney function, sometimes with oliguria.

Differential diagnosis

Fever and severe constitutional disturbance often suggest infection and, until multi-system involvement becomes apparent, much time may be expended in a fruitless search for occult infection.

The concurrence of arthralgia with neurological, cutaneous and renal features may suggest SLE. However, PAN is often a disease of middle-aged men, whereas SLE affects young women. Furthermore, the serological abnormalities of SLE are not usually apparent in PAN.

The purpuric rash needs to be distinguished from that of thrombocytopenia and mixed cryoglobulinaemia (*see* p. 159).

Investigations

Haematological abnormalities of high ESR, leukocytosis and anaemia are non-specific. Eosinophilia occurs in a small percentage of patients with pulmonary involvement. Rheumatoid factors and ANF are found in less than 30% of patients and then in low titre. Serum complement may be low and immune complexes can be demonstrated in the majority of patients. Circulating hepatitis B surface antigen (HB$_s$Ag) can be detected in 10% of cases.

Chest radiographs may show patchy shadows. Arteriography of renal or mesenteric vessels may reveal small aneurysms which are virtually pathognomonic (*Figure 13.1(b)*).

Histological evidence is highly desirable but often difficult to obtain. Muscle and skin biopsy may not yield certain evidence of necrotizing vasculitis. Demonstration of glomerulonephritis in the presence of a multi-system disorder but without serological features of SLE is very suggestive of PAN. Evidence of renal disease may be suggested by proteinuria or microscopic haematuria. Blood creatinine and urea levels should be carefully monitored because renal function can worsen precipitously.

Aetiology

Men are affected four times more frequently than women. There is some evidence that the disease represents a hypersensitivity reaction. Several drugs have been implicated, including penicillin and thiouracil.

The demonstration of immune complexes in the circulation and of immunoglobulins at involved sites suggests a disease of immune complex deposition. This does not preclude a concomitant hypersensitivity response. The presence of HB$_s$Ag in 10% usually occurs in the absence of clinical liver disease. This antigen may participate in the formation of immune complexes. Drug addicts are susceptible to PAN, an association which is sometimes explained by the presence of HB$_s$Ag. Some patients with hairy cell leukaemia also develop polyarteritis.

Pathology

A pan-arteritis occurs in medium sized vessels. Chronic inflammatory cells, polymorphs and eosinophils infiltrate all layers.

Fibrinoid, a purely descriptive histological term, occurs as the intensity of inflammation regresses (fibrinoid necrosis). The lumen becomes occluded and aneurysmal dilatation may be followed by haemorrhage. Tissues supplied by involved vessels are regularly infarcted. Gut, brain, kidneys and skin may exhibit all of these features.

Peripheral neuropathy and mononeuritis are caused by inflammation of the vasa nervorum.

A necrotizing glomerulonephritis occurs in at least 50% of patients. This has no specific histopathological features.

Treatment

This potentially fatal disease requires prompt and aggressive treatment. High dose corticosteroids may be necessary to contain acute symptoms but cyclophosphamide should also be prescribed once the diagnosis is established. This is the immunosuppressive of first choice in PAN.

Hypertension should be treated energetically, preferably with vasodilators. Acute renal failure may demand dialysis. Occasionally renal function does not recover and long-term dialysis or transplantation may need to be contemplated.

Course

The outcome of this disease depends to a large extent on early diagnosis and prompt treatment of the acute illness. Survival of this phase is usually followed by complete recovery. Five-year survival exceeds 75%. Some patients subsequently follow an indolent course in which attempts to modulate treatment are associated with recurrent symptoms. Bowel or myocardial infarction is often a terminal event in these patients.

Other patterns of vasculitis

Wegener's granulomatosis

In this disorder, all the clinical and pathological features of PAN may be combined with granuloma of the sinuses, nasopharynx and lungs. Nasal stuffiness, discharge and respiratory symptoms are associated with radiological evidence of skull bone erosion, clouding of the sinuses and opacities in the lungs. The granulomata comprise necrotic areas surrounded by chronic inflammatory and giant cells. The response to cyclophosphamide treatment is usually good and a previously fatal disease now has an excellent prognosis.

Mixed cryoglobulinaemia

Circulating mixed cryoglobulins (*see* Chapter 3) may be associated with a syndrome of purpuric vasculitis affecting the legs and feet. Arthralgia is usual and peripheral neuropathy an occasional finding. Mixed cryoglobulins may be seen in a range of connective tissue, infectious and lymphoproliferative diseases. Primary Sjögren's syndrome is another associated disorder. In the absence of a recognizable cause, the term 'essential mixed cryoglobulinaemia' is used. Hyperviscosity with arterial thrombosis and retinal haemorrhage is a well documented complication.

Takayasu's arteritis (pulseless disease)

This is very rare in Europe and North America and more commonly affects women in the East. Aortitis and inflammation of the major aortic branches may cause ischaemic pain or major neurological complications. Arthritis, fever and absent peripheral pulses are amongst the more obvious clinical features. Corticosteroid treatment is effective.

Churg- Strauss vasculitis (allergic granulomatous vasculitis)

This rare syndrome comprises lung wheezing, eosinophilia, lung infiltrates (Loffler's syndrome), purpura and peripheral neuropathy. Fibrinoid necrosis of vessels is associated with small, eosinophilic granulomata at sites of involvement.

Henoch Schonlein purpura

Although all age groups may be affected, children are the most susceptible. Arthralgia, peripheral purpura, oedema and abdominal pain may follow an infectious illness. Glomerulonephritis occurs in 50% and sometimes this may be persistent and progressive. The majority of patients have an illness which resolves spontaneously.

Urticarial vasculitis

Recurrent urticaria may be associated with arthralgia, proteinuria and features of angio-neurotic oedema. Isolated urticaria may also have the same constellation of symptoms. This is distinct from the hereditary angio-oedema associated with $C\overline{1}$ inhibitor deficiency.

Other vasculitis

Giant cell arteritis, RA and SLE may each be associated with a necrotizing vasculitis. It is obvious that although vascular inflammation may contribute to the pattern of these diseases, it is not the fundamental pathological event.

Further reading

FAUCI, A. (1979). Vasculitis – new insights amid old enigmas. *Am. J. Med.*, **67,** 916
FAUCI, A. *et al.* (1979). Cyclophosphamide therapy of severe systemic necrotising vasculitis. *N. Engl. J. Med.*, **301,** 235
RONCO, P. *et al.* (1983). Immunopathological studies of polyarthritis nodosa and Wegener's granulomatosis – a report of 43 patients with 51 renal biopsies. *Q. Jl Med.*, **52,** 212

14
Sjögren's syndrome

Inflammation and fibrosis of the salivary and lachrymal glands results in dryness of the eyes and mouth. The syndrome is usually associated with RA, SLE or scleroderma (secondary Sjögren's) but may be an isolated illness (primary Sjögren's).

Symptoms

Dryness of the eyes and mouth (keratoconjunctivitis sicca) may be associated with reduced lubrication of other mucosal surfaces such as the pharynx, trachea and vagina. The eyes may feel sore and are constantly at risk of conjunctivitis. When associated with RA, severe inflammation of the eye may occur. Oropharyngeal dryness leads to difficulty with mastication and swallowing. Laryngeal and tracheal involvement cause hoarseness and vaginal dryness may prevent sexual intercourse. In primary Sjögren's syndrome there may be arthralgia, Raynaud's phenomenon and muscle pain.

Signs

Usually the buccal and conjunctival surfaces do not appear obviously dry but close examination of the eyes with a slit lamp and rose bengal staining reveals punctate keratitis. Scarring and gross ulceration of the cornea are less common.

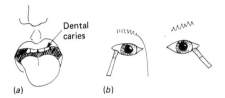

Figure 14.1 Sjögren's syndrome. (a) Dry mouth and tongue, poor dentition; (b) dry eyes being examined by the Schirmer test

Dentition tends to be poor and patients either have multiple caries or are edentulous (*Figure 14.1(a)*). Parotid swelling is usually absent but may be subtle and evidence of RA, SLE or scleroderma should be sought because primary Sjögren's syndrome is a less common disorder.

Differential diagnosis

Keratoconjunctivitis sicca (KCS; sicca syndrome) may occur with ageing and in the absence of local inflammation. This is not Sjögren's syndrome.

Mucosal dryness may be caused by drugs with anticholinergic effects.

Investigations

Clinical suspicion should be followed by a Schirmer test in which strips of standard filter paper are inserted on the lower lids to measure the distance tear secretions move along their length (*Figure 14.1(b)*). A positive test should be followed by slit lamp examination with rose bengal staining. Some academic departments pursue the diagnosis by labial biopsy, salivary flow estimations, sialography and nuclear scanning of the parotid glands.

Elevation of the ESR is common and serological abnormalities may reflect those of an associated connective tissue disease.

In primary Sjögren's syndrome there may be neutropenia, IgM RF, mixed cryoglobulinaemia, speckled staining for ANF and antibodies against the extractable nuclear antigens Ro and La (sometimes called SSA and SSB). These antibodies also occur when Sjögren's syndrome is associated with SLE but not when associated with RA or scleroderma. Some patients with primary Sjögren's have biochemical evidence of renal tubular acidosis.

Aetiology

Women are affected nine times more frequently than men.

The association with illnesses in which immune mechanisms are important points strongly to involvement of the immune system. The range of antibodies reported in both primary and secondary Sjögren's reflects this but gives little indication of why secretory glands should be involved by disparate diseases. Secondary Sjögren's has also been described in primary biliary cirrhosis, graft versus host disease and autoimmune thyroid disease. Primary Sjögren's syndrome is associated with the presence of HLA DR3 and HLA B8. *In vitro* immunoregulatory lymphocyte defects have been recorded in primary Sjögren's and delayed skin sensitivity is also impaired.

Pathology

Salivary and lachrymal glands are infiltrated with both B and T lymphocytes in varying proportions. The T cells are mainly of the helper inducer class. Acinar disruption and fibrosis subsequently occur.

Treatment

Artificial tears and saliva can be prescibed but are less than adequate replacements for a continuous flow of the natural secretions. Oral bromhexine may stimulate tear production but is of uncertain value. Surgical occlusion of the nasolachrymal duct may help the retention of a tear film. Corticosteroids and immunosuppressive drugs have no proven value but are occasionally beneficial.

Course

This is a disagreeable illness but not all patients experience relentless worsening of their symptoms. Spontaneous improvement occasionally occurs.

A small number of patients develop gross enlargement of salivary and cervical lymph nodes or pulmonary infiltrates. These are characterized by dense accumulations of lymphocytes and the picture is called pseudolymphoma. In addition to this benign complication, patients with Sjögren's syndrome (especially primary disease) are susceptible to malignant lymphoproliferative disorders such as Hodgkin's disease and Waldenstrom's macroglobulinaemia.

Further reading

EDITORIAL (1984). Primary and secondary Sjögren's syndrome. *Lancet*, **2,** 730
MOUTSOPOULOS, H. *et al.* (1980). Sjögren's syndrome (sicca syndrome): current issues. *Ann. Intern. Med.*, **92,** 212

15
Rheumatic disorders of children

Joint and musculoskeletal pain in children has many possible causes other than chronic arthritis. Trauma, viral infections and malignant diseases are a few of the disorders which may cause joint symptoms.

Juvenile chronic arthritis (JCA)

This is defined as joint inflammation which persists for at least three months in children of less than 16 years of age and for which there is no other obvious cause. Three major clinical patterns are recognized: systemic onset, pauciarticular disease and poly-articular disease.

Systemic onset

This affects children of any age, and boys slightly more often than girls. A swinging fever may coincide with a pink, transient rash on the trunk and limbs, often occurring in the evening. Polyarthritis of small and large joints; lymph node, liver and spleen enlargement; pleurisy and pericarditis are all common manifestations. Arthritis tends to persist when other features have regressed.

Investigations may reveal anaemia, leukocytosis and negative tests for rheumatoid factor (RF) and ANF. Radiology may reveal joint erosions and one-third of patients develop severely disabling joint destruction. Although rare, the disease may occur in adults.

Pauciarticular disease

A few joints are involved and these are most often knees, ankles and wrists. Patients can be further categorized into two subgroups:

1. Patients with the equivalent of adult ankylosing spondylitis. These are mainly older boys who have predominant involvement of the lower limbs. Spinal symptoms are absent but clinical and radiological evidence of sacroiliitis may be apparent in adolescence and some patients develop ankylosing spondylitis as they emerge from childhood. Acute iritis occurs occasionally.
    Laboratory tests usually reveal elevation of ESR and negative tests for RF and ANF. HLA B27 is found in 80%. Radiology of the sacroiliac joints is unhelpful until late adolescence because the normal appearance in childhood resembles that of sacroiliitis in the adult.
2. The other group tends to affect young girls and the knees, elbows and wrists are frequently involved. This disease is characterized by a chronic and insidious form of iridocyclitis which may cause blindness, even when treated. This is distinct from the acute iritis described above.
    The most striking serological abnormality is a positive ANF test which occurs in 50%. Radiographs reveal little cartilage loss and few erosions. Ankylosis of the wrists may be a late sequel. The outlook for these children is generally excellent.

Polyarticular disease

This symmetrical arthritis involves small and large joints. Girls are affected ten times more frequently than boys. Children of all ages may be susceptible, although patients with positive RF tests tend to be older.

Radiographs may reveal features identical to those of adult rheumatoid arthritis. Children with positive RF tests tend to fare worse and their arthritis usually persists into adulthood.

Treatment

Rest, splints, muscle exercises, salicylates and other anti-inflammatory drugs form the basis of management. Second-line agents such as sodium aurothiomalate, D-penicillamine, antimalarials and corticosteroids may be used in more severe patterns of JCA with a measure of success. The dose of drugs has to be related to the size of the patient. Intra-articular corticosteroids have a limited place because needles may terrorize children to an extent that rapport is lost. The role of surgery is similar to that of adult RA and joint replacements are performed with increasing frequency. All children and especially those with pauciarticular disease require regular slit lamp examination of the eyes for the early detection of iritis. Prompt use of local and systemic corticosteroids may preserve sight.

Adequate compensation for lost schooling should be arranged through home or hospital tuition.

Course

Severe JCA causes stunting of growth and precocious epiphyseal fusion. Consequent stigmata may include under-development of the mandible (micrognathia) and ankylosis of cervical vertebrae (*Figure 15.1*). Corticosteroids may contribute to retardation of growth although this risk is lessened with alternate day therapy.

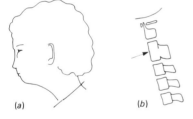

Figure 15.1 Juvenile chronic arthritis. (a) Micrognathia – under-development of the mandible; (b) fusion of the third and fourth cervical vertebrae.

The majority of children with JCA have a good outlook and lead normal adult lives. Pauciarticular disease carries the best prognosis and seropositive polyarthritis the worst.

Rheumatic fever

This is now exceptionally rare in Western Europe and North America but is common in communities which are poor or undeveloped.

Classically, arthritis affects large or small joints 10–21 days after a sore throat and symptoms migrate from one joint to another.

Fever is usual and a characteristic rash, erythema marginatum, may be a feature. Small nodules often develop in clusters over pressure points.

Tachycardia, pericarditis, heart murmurs, cardiomegaly, heart failure or a prolonged P–R interval on ECG are evidence of cardiac involvement. The features of Sydenham's chorea may develop, comprising involuntary, purposeless and rapid movements of the extremities.

Although a history of a sore throat is not always obtained, a rising titre of anti-streptolysin O or other anti-streptococcal antibodies confirms the close association between group A streptococcal infection and rheumatic fever. Patients who develop the disease tend to have higher titres than those with infection but no rheumatic fever. It is suspected, but not proven, that there is a genetic predisposition. The reason for the disappearance of rheumatic fever may, in part, be related to the diminished frequency of streptococcal infection in advanced societies, but reduced virulence of the organism may also be contributory.

Cross-reactivity between anti-streptococcal A antibodies and human tissues, including heart muscle, has been shown. These findings may or may not have pathogenetic significance.

The most characteristic pathological finding is the Aschoff nodule. This occurs in the myocardium but subcutaneous nodules have a similar appearance. Essentially they are areas of fibrinoid with a variable cellular surrounding of lymphocytes and histiocytes. Inflammatory cells may infiltrate the myocardium and pericardium and myocardial necrosis may occur. An endocarditis is manifest by exudate on the valve cusps.

Treatment

Bed rest and a weight-related anti-inflammatory dose of a salicylate preparation are conventional. Corticosteroids may be given when heart failure threatens, and penicillin prophylaxis against further streptococcal pharyngitis should continue until adulthood.

Course

Evidence of arthritis and carditis recedes over several weeks or months. Chorea follows a similar time course but occasionally persists for more than a year.

Later development of clinically significant rheumatic heart disease is unpredictable. Penicillin prophylaxis should nevertheless be recommended for those with a history of rheumatic carditis who later undergo surgery or dental procedures. Persistent joint deformities occasionally occur and are called Jaccoud's arthropathy.

Common non-inflammatory causes of knee pain

Osteochondritis dissecans

Recurrent pain and effusion of a knee may be associated with necrosis and subsequent loosening of a small segment of femoral condyle bone. Diagnosis can be difficult because radiographs may

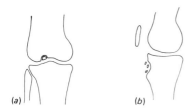

Figure 15.2   Causes of knee pain in children. (a) Osteochondritis dissecans; (b) Osgood Schlatter's disease

be initially normal. A bone scan may reveal the defect but if the fragment eventually separates a bone defect and a loose body should become obvious radiologically (*Figure 15.2(a)*).

Failure to remove the loose body may cause recurrent locking of the joint and osteoarthritis in adulthood.

Chondromalacia patellae

This diagnosis may represent several different pathologies of the anterior compartment of the knee. The patient is usually a physically robust child or adolescent with intermittent pain of one or both knees. Symptoms are accentuated by climbing stairs and, on examination, pain is reproduced by compression of the patella against the femoral condyles. Joint effusions are not a feature and patello-femoral crepitus is often found but may also be a feature of asymptomatic joints.

Roughening of the retropatellar cartilage may account for some cases but others have no clearly defined pathology.

Treatment is best confined to symptomatic measures, quadriceps strengthening and avoidance of relevant activities. Symptoms may take several years to disappear. There is no relationship between this syndrome and osteoarthritis and parents may require reassurance. Surgery should be avoided if possible.

Trauma

Children and young adults commonly engage in sport. Joint pain, especially of the knee, may be attributed to a sporting injury although such a history may be misleading (*see* Chapter 11). Mechanical derangements such as torn menisci can occur in children.

Osgood Schlatter's disease

Pain may on inspection be derived from the infrapatellar region at the insertion of the ligamentum patellae. There may be associated swelling and tenderness. Symptoms are caused by separation of the immature epiphysis from the tibia (*Figure 15.2(b)*). Restricted activity within the limits of pain is followed by improvement over a period of months.

Other causes of childhood joint pain

Perthes disease

This causes a limp with hip or knee pain between the ages of 5 and 11. Boys are affected more frequently than girls. Radiographs may show initial widening of the joint space followed by sclerosis, flattening and irregularity of the femoral head.

Treatment now tends to be confined to simple observation without calipers or other measures. Restoration of the femoral head may occur over 1–4 years.

Scheuermann's disease

This is most often seen in early adolescence. Dorsal back pain may be associated with a kyphosis and characteristic radiological features (*see* Chapter 6 and *Figure 6.1(e)*). Symptoms settle within 1–2 years but a kyphosis usually persists.

Miscellaneous

Most of the rheumatic disorders seen in adults may also affect children. Joint sepsis, viral arthritis, reactive arthritis, enteric arthritis, psoriatic arthropathy, SLE and scleroderma have all been described.

Childhood dermatomyositis is distinct from the disorder seen in adults. A facial rash similar to that of SLE may be associated with a rash in the distribution of adult dermatomyositis. Clinical and laboratory evidence of myositis varies in severity. Recovery may be followed by widespread subcutaneous and muscle calcification with wasting. The skin may come to resemble that of scleroderma and skin ulceration often occurs at sites of calcification. Corticosteroid treatment is effective in the acute phase of the illness.

Malignant diseases such as lymphoma, leukaemia and neuroblastoma may present with limb and joint pain. Signs of joint inflammation may occur with leukaemia.

Further reading

ANSELL, B. (1983). Arthritis in young children. *Br. Med. J.,* **286,** 1917

ARNETT, F. *et al.* (1980). Juvenile onset chronic arthritis – clinical and roenterographic features of a unique HLA B27 subset. *Am. J. Med.,* **69,** 369

ELKON, K. *et al.* (1982). Adult onset Stills disease – 20 year follow up and further studies of patients with active disease. *Arthritis Rheum.,* **25,** 647

16
Soft tissue inflammation

This constitutes a range of common rheumatic complaints some of which are caused by trauma or overuse. They are all disorders which can be disabling and their treatment should be within the scope of every physician.

The painful shoulder

Painful shoulder movement may be the consequence of inflammation involving one or more tendons of the rotator cuff muscles. These are the supraspinatus, infraspinatus, teres minor, long head of triceps, subscapularis and long head of biceps (*Figure 16.1*).

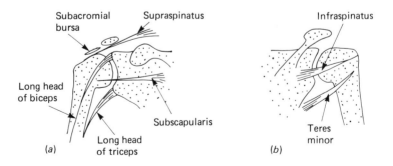

Figure 16.1   Muscles of the rotator cuff: (a) anterior; (b) posterior

Supraspinatus tendonitis

This is associated with a painful arc on abduction of the arm, coinciding with movement of the inflamed segment beneath the acromion and the coraco–acromial ligament. This clinical picture may be associated with radiological evidence of tendon calcification. In calcific tendonitis, pain may be acute, severe and associated with warmth and swelling of the shoulder. Calcium hydroxyapatite may be shed into the sub-acromial bursa which also becomes inflamed.

Bicipital tendonitis

This can be distinguished by pain on resisted forearm flexion and tenderness of the long head of the biceps.

Precise diagnosis of inflammation involving other rotator cuff muscle is more difficult. Pain which is increased by resisted muscle contraction and tenderness at sites of insertion may help localization. When symptoms cannot be easily attributed to a single muscle, the diagnosis 'rotator cuff syndrome' is appropriate.

Adhesive capsulitis (frozen shoulder)

If neglected, pain in one muscle tendon may be followed by inflammation and adherence of the joint capsule to all the rotator cuff muscles. This causes painful restriction of movement in every direction and is termed 'adhesive capsulitis' or 'frozen shoulder'.

Adhesive capsulitis is more common amongst diabetics and may be associated with anticonvulsant treatment. In addition to local causes it may follow referred pain from ischaemic heart and gall bladder disease, cervical spondylosis, hemiplegia and mastectomy.

Distinction from cervical spine disease, polymyalgia rheumatica, and RA is usually possible. Osteoarthritis occasionally involves the shoulders. Painful disintegration of the joint is occasionally seen and the finding of calcium hydroxyapatite crystals in the joint fluid of such patients has prompted the suggestion that the crystals are pathogenetic (Milwaukee shoulder). Painful wasting of the deltoid may be due to neuralgic amyotrophy, an acute, benign illness possibly caused by viral infection.

In general, haematological and biochemical investigations are normal in adhesive capsulitis. Radiographs may show some roughening of the humeral insertion of rotator cuff muscles and narrowing of the space between humeral head and the acromion.

Treatment

Isolated rotator cuff tendonitis may remit spontaneously or be modified by anti-inflammatory drugs. Persistent symptoms are often responsive to corticosteroid injections placed in the relevant tendon. When several tendons seem to be implicated (rotator cuff syndrome), injections into the sub-acromial space and joint cavity are often effective. The same approach can be attempted for adhesive capsulitis (*Figure 16.2*).

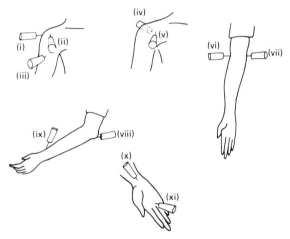

Figure 16.2 Injection sites for soft tissue lesions of the upper limb: (i) lateral approach to sub-acromial space; (ii) anterior approach to sub-acromial space; (iii) long head of biceps; (iv) posterior approach to gleno–humeral joint; (v) anterior approach to gleno–humeral joint; (vi) lateral epicondylitis; (vii) medial epicondylitis; (viii) olecranon bursitis; (ix) De Quervain's tenosynovitis; (x) carpal tunnel syndrome; (xi) finger flexor tenosynovitis or trigger finger

Physical treatment such as short wave diathermy may reduce pain and exercises may lessen the risk of adhesive capsulitis or help restore movement when this has already developed.

Course

Single or limited tendon involvement usually remits completely in response to these measures. Adhesive capsulitis may respond only partially and restricted movement may persist for at least two years after treatment.

Epicondylitis

Symptoms of lateral epicondylitis (tennis elbow) develop after prolonged or unaccustomed use of an arm in repetitive movement or gripping. Pain is situated over the lateral aspect of the elbow and in the forearm. Tenderness may be maximal over or in the proximity of the lateral epicondyle. Pain is accentuated by gripping and by resisted dorsiflexion of the wrist.

Epicondylitis represents an example of an enthesopathy, a term used to describe lesions of ligament or muscle attachments to bone and periosteum. In this instance, symptoms arise at the origin of the wrist dorsiflexors.

An analagous but less common picture occurs on the medial aspect of the elbow. This is due to an enthesopathy of the medial epicondyle at the origin of the wrist flexor muscles (golfer's elbow).

Treatment

Recognition and modification of the activity responsible for symptoms may help. An injection of hydrocortisone into the site of maximal tenderness is the best therapeutic option (*Figure 16.2(vi)* and *(vii)*). Physical treatment such as ultrasound may be beneficial.

Course

Epicondylitis is often resistant to treatment and tends to recur, usually because the offending activity is related to employment or some pleasurable leisure pursuit.

Olecranon bursitis

Painful swelling of the olecranon bursa is usually caused by trauma. When associated with inflammatory joint disease such as RA it is also likely to be traumatic in aetiology because patients tend to use elbows for supporting the upper part of their bodies rather than their painful hands. In gout, olecranon bursitis is caused by crystals within the bursa. Occasionally, the bursitis is due to infection.

Aspiration of the bursa usually yields blood or xanthochromic fluid. Crystals may be seen in gout and organisms cultured in septic bursitis. A hydrocortisone injection may speed resolution of very painful bursitis (*Figure 16.2(viii)*). Persistent or recurrent inflammation may require surgical excision of the bursa.

De Quervain's tenosynovitis

Inflammation of tendons and their sheaths may occur at any site but is most frequent in the hands. Involvement of the pollicis tendons may cause severe pain, swelling and crepitus along their lower course in the forearm and the base of the thumb. The onset is acute and is usually associated with some obvious overuse activity. Symptoms often resolve spontaneously within days. Persistent discomfort usually responds to a single hydrocortisone injection (*Figure 16.2(ix)*). Longer acting and more potent corticosteroid injections such as methylprednisolone may cause skin and subcutaneous atrophy when used to treat lesions near the surface (epicondylitis, bursitis, tenosynovitis).

Carpal tunnel syndrome

Compression of the median nerve at the wrist causes pain, paraesthesiae and numbness of the fingers which is characteristically worse at night and in the early morning. Pain may be referred proximally into the forearm and occasionally the upper arm. The sensory symptoms which patients describe may not correspond with the median nerve distribution. Percussion of the carpal tunnel may reproduce pain or paraesthesiae (Tinel's sign). There may be weakness and wasting of the thenar eminence and reduced sensation in one or more of the digits supplied by the median nerve.

Distinction from cervical spondylosis is sometimes difficult. Wasting of the thenar eminence is most commonly due to OA of the thumb but when associated with interosseus wasting may also be due to peripheral neuropathy or T1 nerve root compression. Pancoast tumour must be excluded if signs and investigations fail to confirm median nerve compression. Nerve conduction studies are helpful when there is diagnostic uncertainty.

Any condition which causes narrowing of the carpal tunnel may result in the syndrome. Thus, fluid retention in pregnancy or increased local swelling due to obesity, hypothyroidism, osteo-arthritis, inflammatory joint disese or acromegaly may each be responsible.

Treatment

Severe symptoms are best treated by injecting the carpal tunnel with corticosteroid even if a correctible underlying cause can be identified (*Figure 16.2(x)*). Most patients obtain at least some relief from this procedure. Rest of the wrist in a splint at night may also be helpful.

If these measures fail, surgical decompression is warranted. This is a simple procedure which may be undertaken as an out patient.

Flexor tenosynovitis or trigger finger

Tenosynovitis may affect the flexor tendons of the fingers and usually has the same aetiology, treatment and course as De Quervain's tenosynovitis. Chronic or recurrent inflammation may cause progressive narrowing of the tendon sheath and a restricted range of finger extension. This is a common observation in RA but is also a feature of some occupations in which the palms are subjected to repeated trauma or use. It should not be confused with Dupuytren's contracture, which is due to fibrosis and contraction of the palmar fascia.

The narrowed tendon sheath is sometimes associated with an inflammatory nodule in the tendon. This combination may cause obstruction of free movement and an inability to extend a flexed digit unless additional force is applied. Release of the tendon may be associated with acute pain and a click. A corticosteroid injection into the involved tendon sheath may be curative but surgical release is sometimes required (*Figure 16.2(xi)*).

Tietze's syndrome

Painful, tender costochondral junctions may be seen in RA and ankylosing spondylitis but may also occur as an isolated phenomenon. Swelling was a feature originally described by Tietze but is not commonly seen. The aetiology is obscure and the symptoms tend to remit spontaneously. Local infiltration with corticosteroid may help.

Groin strain

Enthesopathies around the hip may involve the ilio–femoral or pubo–femoral ligaments and the pelvic attachments of the adductors and pectineus muscles. Pain may limit physical activity

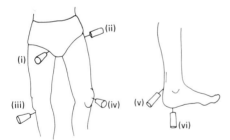

Figure 16.3 Injection sites for soft tissue lesions of the lower limb: (i) groin strain; (ii) trochanteric bursitis; (iii) infra-patellar bursitis; (iv) pre-patellar bursitis; (v) para-tendon region in Achilles tendonitis; (vi) plantar fasciitis

but does not impede walking. Discomfort may be increased by resisted hip flexion or adduction and there may be tenderness over the adductor tubercle. The symptoms are usually the outcome of excessive running.

Treatment is notoriously difficult. Physical remedies, anti-inflammatory drugs and corticosteroid injections have only a slight chance of success (*Figure 16.3(i)*). Symptoms may resolve after a prolonged period of months or even years.

Ischial and trochanteric bursitis

Pain and tenderness over the ischia (weaver's bottom) or greater trochanter may be due to bursitis at these sites. Corticosteroid injections are the best treatment (*Figure 16.3(ii)*).

Bursitis of the knee

Pain and swelling around the knee is sometimes due to inflammation of the pre-patellar (housemaid's knee) or infra-patellar (clergyman's knee) bursae. The cause is usually trauma although gout and sepsis may be responsible. The findings and treatment are those outlined for olecranon bursitis (*see* p. 175). Occasionally, pain on the medial aspect of the tibia beneath the sartorius muscle is due to an anserine bursitis. Swelling is not obvious and an injection of steroid into the site of tenderness is usually adequate treatment (*Figure 16.3(iii)* and *(iv)*).

Achilles tendonitis

Painful thickening of the Achilles tendon may follow prolonged running, especially on a hard surface. As with soft tissue inflammation at other sites, symptoms are usually worse in the morning. Rest, ultrasound treatment and para-tendon injections of steroid may help (*Figure 16.3(v)*). Corticosteroid injected into the tendon may predispose to its rupture and should be avoided.

Shin splints and tibial stress fractures

Pain over the anterior tibial compartment may occur in runners. Some cases are due to tibial stress fractures but others have muscle-derived pain of obscure aetiology. There is no effective treatment other than restricted activity.

Plantar fasciitis

Heel pain which is characteristically worse in the morning may occur in subjects who do a lot of standing or walking. Tenderness is the only sign and a radiograph may show a calcaneal spur although this may also be seen in painless heels. Plantar fasciitis is a common feature of some inflammatory joint diseases, evidence for which must be sought.

Treatment comprises a soft heel pad, an elevated shoe heel or a corticosteroid injection into the painful site (*Figure 16.3(vi)*).

Further reading

BLAND, J. *et al.* (1977). The painful shoulder. Sem. *Arthritis Rheum.*, **7,** 21

McCARTY, D. *et al.* (1981). Milwaukee shoulder. *Arthritis Rheum.*, **24,** 464

OZDOGAN, H. and YAZICI, H. (1984). The efficacy of local steroid injections in idiopathic carpal tunnel syndrome: a double blind study. *Br. J. Rheum.*, **23,** 272

17
Metabolic and endocrine causes of joint pain

Metabolic

Diabetes mellitus

There are number of clinical associations between joint pain and diabetes.

1. Painful feet associated with diabetic peripheral neuropathy may be wrongly attributed to arthritis of the toes. The painful quadriceps wasting of diabetic amyotrophy may be mistaken for hip or lumbar spine disease. Carpal tunnel syndrome is more common, possibly because peripheral nerves are more susceptible to injury in diabetes. Diabetic radiculopathy may simulate lumbar disc protrusion.
2. Diabetic peripheral neuropathy is now the most common cause of Charcot joints. The hind foot, ankle and knees are the most vulnerable (*Figure 17.1*).

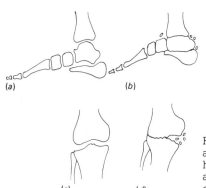

(a)   (b)

(c)   (d)

Figure 17.1 Charcot joints in diabetes: (a) normal foot; (b) ankle and hind foot in diabetic neuropathic arthropathy; (c) normal knee; (d) disorganized knee

181

3. Cysts and erosions of the metatarsals are occasionally seen (diabetic osteolysis). These may be confused with gout, RA or other inflammatory diseases.
4. There is a strong association between adhesive capsulitis of the shoulder and diabetes. Blood glucose estimations should be performed in all patients with this disorder.
5. It has been claimed that osteoarthritis is more common amongst diabetics.
6. Diffuse idiopathic skeletal hyperostosis (DISH, Forestier's disease) is more frequently seen.
7. Some patients with insulin dependent, and occasionally non-insulin dependent, diabetes develop tightening of the skin over their fingers, resembling scleroderma (cheiroarthropathy).

Haemochromatosis

Joint pain occurs in 50% of patients with primary haemochromatosis. Increased iron stores are found in the synovium as well as the heart, liver, pancreas and other organs. It is not clear how iron in the joint initiates the characteristic arthropathy.

The fingers are the most frequent site of involvement but arthralgia may be widespread. Tenderness and slight swelling of the second and third metacarpophalangeal (MCP) joints are the most consistent findings (*Figure 17.2*). Acute pain and swelling of large joints occurs occasionally due to pseudogout.

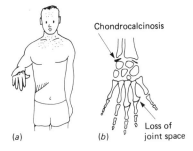

Chondrocalcinosis

Loss of joint space

(a)   (b)

Figure 17.2 Haemochromatosis: (a) man with hepatomegaly, pigmentation and arthritis of the second and third MCP joints; (b) radiograph showing chondrocalcinosis of the wrist and loss of joint space confined to the second and third MCP joints

Radiographs usually demonstrate loss of joint space of the second and third MCP joints and chondrocalcinosis of the wrists, knees and other sites. Occasionally, the chondrocalcinosis is associated with a destructive arthritis.

Treatment of the increased iron stores by phlebotomy does not seem to influence the joint symptoms.

Ochronosis (alkaptonuria)

The rare deficiency of homogentisate oxidase leads to accumulation of homogentisic acid in the body. The urine turns black on standing and cartilage may become similarly stained. The pinnae, nasal cartilage and sclerae may be visibly darkened. The pigment also causes alterations to the physical properties of cartilage which in the spine and joints degenerates prematurely. Precocious osteoarthritis of the spine and peripheral joints is usually associated with calcification of the intervertebral discs and articular hyaline cartilage.

Hypercholesterolaemia

Type II hyperlipoproteinaemia is often familial and associated with a high serum cholesterol, xanthelesma and xanthomata. Some patients experience recurrent episodes of acute arthritis affecting large or small joints. Xanthomata on the elbows or Achilles tendons may be mistaken for gouty tophi or rheumatoid nodules in the presence of joint pain. The cause of the arthritis is obscure. Cholesterol crystals can be seen in the joint effusions of this and several other disorders and are not thought to be of pathogenetic significance.

Endocrine

Acromegaly

Overgrowth of cartilage causes a radiographic widening of joint spaces, a feature which may be of diagnostic value. The enlarged skeleton and thickened cartilage may alter the normal mechanical alignment of joint surfaces, causing precocious osteoarthritis. The prevalence of chondrocalcinosis is also increased. Carpal tunnel syndrome may result from increased bone beneath the flexor retinaculum. Diffuse idiopathic skeletal hyperostosis may occur and the spine may also appear osteoporotic. Backache and spinal stiffness are common clinical features.

Hyperparathyroidism

This topic is discussed in Chapter 7 (see p.71). In brief, proximal myopathy, pseudogout, chondrocalcinosis and bone pain constitute the musculoskeletal manifestations.

Primary hypoparathyroidism

This rare disease usually presents with muscle weakness due to hypocalcaemia. Stiffness of the spine due to longitudinal ligament ossification has been described. The radiological picture may resemble diffuse idiopathic skeletal hyperostosis.

Hypothyroidism

The association of hypothyroidism with carpal tunnel syndrome is well known. Not every patient who is deficient in thyroxine presents with classical symptoms and signs. It is an important cause of vague musculoskeletal pain and stiffness and symptoms can resemble polymyalgia rheumatica and RA.

A proximal myopathy may account for some pain. Weakness is not pronounced but the diagnosis may be confirmed by electromyography. Serum creatine phosphokinase (CPK) is often elevated in hypothyroidism even in the absence of clinical myopathy.

Small joint effusions may be seen but these are usually incidental. Non-inflammatory effusions in hypothyroidism tend to be very viscous. There is an increased frequency of chondrocalcinosis. In severe hypothyroidism the skin may become oedematous and resemble that of early scleroderma.

Further reading

CRISP, A. and HEATHCOTE, J. (1984). Connective tissue abnormalities in diabetes mellitus. *J. Roy. Coll. Phys.*, **18**, 132

HAMILTON, E. (1981). The natural history of arthritis in idiopathic haemochromatosis – progression of the clinical and radiological features over 10 years. *Q. Jl. Med.*, **50**, 321

18
Miscellaneous disorders and disease associations

Agammaglobulinaemia

Both the X-linked disease of children and that of adults (common variable immunodeficiency) may be associated with a polyarthritis which resembles RA but neither joint deformities nor erosions occur. Symptoms respond to injections of gamma globulin.

Alcohol

Ethanol abuse is a common yet poorly recognized cause of musculoskeletal pain. It may be manifest by any of the following:

1. Proximal myopathy with vague pain and stiffness or more florid features, including weakness;
2. Pain and paraesthesiae due to peripheral neuropathy;
3. Acute arthritis due to gout;
4. Bone or joint pain due to avascular necrosis;
5. Rib or spinal pain due to fractures following drunken falls.

Algodystrophy (Sudeck's atrophy)

This is a poorly understood phenomenon which affects a hand or foot and, less commonly, other skeletal sites. There is often a history of injury with delayed recovery. The extremity is often swollen, painful, shiny, discoloured and moist. The shoulder hand syndrome is a specific example in which an adhesive capsulitis is associated with algodystrophy of the hand. It is presumed that some disorder of vasomotor control contributes to the findings. Sympathetic blockade is sometimes helpful but the problem can be protracted and resistant to all measures.

Amyloidosis

Amyloid is an amorphous staining material which under electron microscopy is seen to be comprised of rigid, non-branching fibrils and a pentagonal unit (P component). The fibrillar protein may be composed of amyloid A protein (AA) which resembles and is probably derived from serum AA protein (SAA). The latter behaves like an acute phase reactant and is elevated in RA (see Chapter 5) and other inflammatory, infectious or neoplastic diseases. The fibrillar protein may also be derived from immunoglobulin light chains (see Chapter 3). Amyloid is seen at various sites as an intercellular deposit. Traces occur regularly in the heart, pancreas and blood vessels of elderly subjects.

Several patterns of clinical amyloidosis occur:

1. Primary amyloid is seen in middle aged and elderly patients, men more often than women. Peripheral neuropathy, purpura, macroglossia, heart failure, nephrotic syndrome, carpal tunnel syndrome and arthritis may occur. The arthritis is characterized by swelling of the shoulders. Usually there is an increased monoclonal immunoglobulin in the serum and evidence of plasma cell dyscrasia in the marrow. Some people classify the primary amyloidosis of multiple myeloma separately. The fibrillar protein in these cases is related to serum immunoglobulin light chains (AL). Treatment is that of the underlying plasma cell disorder.

2. Secondary amyloid, comprising AA fibrillar protein, is a sequel to chronic diseases. Rheumatoid arthritis is the most frequent cause but other inflammatory joint disorders may have the same outcome, including juvenile chronic arthritis. Tuberculosis, leprosy and lymphoma are other worldwide causes. The clinical features are nephrotic syndrome and hepato-splenomegaly, although it is recognized that the amyloid may be found in the

rectal and gingival mucosa and subcutaneous tissues. All these sites may provide histological confirmation of the diagnosis. There is no really effective treatment apart from suppression of the underlying disease.

3. Familial amyloidosis has several distinct patterns which result in either peripheral neuropathy, cardiomyopathy or nephrotic syndrome. Familial Mediterranean fever is the best known of these. Semitic people are the most likely victims of the illness, which comprises recurrent episodes of fever, pleurisy, peritonitis, arthritis and renal disease. Colchicine may reduce the frequency of acute symptoms but does not necessarily influence the progression of renal amyloid deposition.

Avascular necrosis

Small areas of bone infarction may occur when small arteries are occluded in decompression sickness (seen frequently in North Sea divers and tunnel workers), alcoholics, sickle cell disease, corticosteroid treatment, pancreatic disease, fractured femoral neck and possibly gout. No cause can be identified in a proportion of patients.

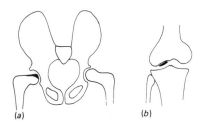

Figure 18.1 Avascular necrosis: (a) flattening and sclerosis of the femoral head; (b) sclerosis and separation of a segment of femoral condyle at the knee

Lesions often occur at the end of long bones with consequent necrosis and collapse of joint surfaces. The femoral and humeral heads and femoral condyles are common sites of involvement (*Figure 18.1*).

Corticosteroids account for the frequency of avascular necrosis in SLE and transplant patients. Pancreatic disease may cause liberation of fat droplets which can obstruct small vessels.

Calcific periarthritis

Deposition of calcium hydroxyapatite in the joint capsule of small and large joints may be associated with a clinical picture of recurrent, acute arthritis. There is no obvious metabolic disturbance and the condition is distinct from pseudogout.

Charcot joints

Loss of pain and positional sense in a joint predisposes to gross internal derangement. Originally described in association with syphylitic tabes dorsalis, it is now more commonly seen in diabetic peripheral neuropathy (*see* p. 181). Other causes are leprosy and syringomyelia in which the spine, shoulders, elbows and fingers may be affected. Pronounced and relatively painless deformities occur and seem to cause little disability. Radiographs may show total joint disruption with loose bodies and chondrocalcinosis (*see Figure 17.1*).

Surgical treatment should be avoided because arthrodesis often fails despite prolonged immobilization, and joint replacement is invariably disastrous.

Erythema nodosum

The painful rash of erythema nodosum usually occurs on the legs where it is often associated with painful swelling of the ankles and, less commonly, the knees. Arthralgia and stiffness may be widespread. The painful swelling of the ankles may represent a periarthritis rather than a true synovitis (*Figure 18.2*).

Erythema nodosum has several causes including sarcoidosis, streptococcal infection, tuberculosis, inflammatory bowel disease and drugs. Articular symptoms are unrelated to the aetiology of the rash.

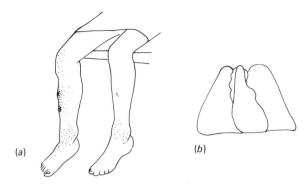

(a)   (b)

Figure 18.2   Erythema nodosum: (a) rash affecting right leg more than left with arthritis of right knee and both ankles, cellulitis and extensive oedema of the right leg and foot; (b) hilar and paratracheal lymph node enlargement of associated sarcoidosis

Fibrositis

Patients with degenerative disease of the cervical or lumbar spine may develop tender sites distal to the spine. It is thought that a similar mechanism may account for pain and tenderness at several predictable trigger areas of the trunk and extremities in patients without spinal symptoms. A disturbed pattern of sleep is a frequent finding in such patients, who may also display obsessional traits of personality.

Haemophilic arthropathy

The arthritis of haemophilia can cause permanent disability. Knees, ankles and other large joints are the most vulnerable. Acute haemarthrosis is recognized by severe pain, warmth and swelling. Recurrent bleeds cause synovial proliferation and irreversible cartilage damage. The joint may become unstable, deformed and persistently swollen by effusion.

Radiographs of the knee may show typical widening of the femoral condyles and the tibial spines. There may be progressive loss of cartilage, subchondral cysts and changes of secondary OA.

Acute bleeds should be treated promptly by rest, splintage and Factor VIII replacement. Anti-inflammatory drugs should be avoided but joint aspiration may relieve the pain of a distended joint capsule. Synovectomy may slow progression since it is felt that chronic joint symptoms may be partly due to synovial proliferation.

Hypertrophic osteoarthropathy

Any illness which causes clubbing may also cause the associated syndrome of joint pain and periosteal new bone formation. The most common precipitating disease is bronchial carcinoma. Joints and juxta-articular bone may be tender at sites of periositis but a true synovitis also occurs and may resemble RA.

Hypermobility

Children have relatively supple joints, the mobility of which decreases with age. Some adults may exhibit an exaggerated range of joint movement of one or several joints (*Figure 18.3*). Occasionally this can be linked to an underlying disorder of collagen such as Ehlers Danlos and Marfan's syndromes. Other so

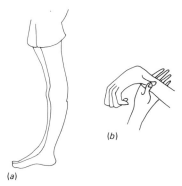

(a)

(b)

Figure 18.3 Hypermobility: (a) hyper-extensibility of the knee (genu recurvatum); (b) demonstrating hypermobility of the thumb

far unrecognized abnormalities of collagen may account for some patients with widespread hypermobility. There may be an association with mitral valve prolapse (floppy valve). It is thought that arthralgia and joint injury are more likely to arise in subjects with generalized hypermobility.

Liver disease

There are a number of clinical associations between liver and joint disorders:

1. Mild hepatic dysfunction may occur in several joint diseases including RA, polymyalgia rheumatica and SLE.
2. Liver enzyme abnormalities may be provoked by salicylates in SLE and juvenile chronic arthritis. Other anti-inflammatory drugs may cause liver dysfunction in any disease.
3. Autoimmune liver disease (primary biliary cirrhosis, chronic active hepatitis) may be associated with Sjögren's syndrome. Primary biliary cirrhosis occasionally occurs with scleroderma and there is some evidence that this liver disease may be associated with a specific arthritis. In chronic active hepatitis, an arthritis, rash, pleurisy, pericarditis or glomerulonephritis may be seen. The picture may resemble SLE and this association evoked the now defunct expression 'lupoid hepatitis'. In chronic active hepatitis, even without these features, there may be a positive test for ANF. In chronic active hepatitis antibody against smooth muscle is often present, and in primary biliary cirrhosis the serological hallmark is mitochondrial antibody.
4. Evidence of liver disorder, osteoarthritis and chondrocalcinosis should always arouse suspicion of haemochromatosis.
5. Gout is commonly associated with alcoholic liver disease.
6. Arthritis may precede jaundice in infectious hepatitis.

Osteomyelitis

Bone infection may simulate arthritis when it arises near a joint. A sympathetic synovial effusion may occur, suggesting that there is primary joint pathology. This diagnostic problem can be particularly difficult in children.

Osteochondritis

Several disorders which are aetiologically unrelated are often described under this heading because they affect the immature skeleton. Thus, Perthes, Scheuermann's and Osgood Schlatter's diseases (*see* Chapter 15) may be categorized together.

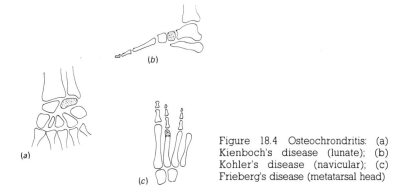

Figure 18.4 Osteochrondritis: (a) Kienboch's disease (lunate); (b) Kohler's disease (navicular); (c) Frieberg's disease (metatarsal head)

Pain and tenderness associated with radiological evidence of bone deformity and sclerosis may arise in children or young adults over the tarsal navicular (Kohler's disease), the second or less commonly the third, fourth or fifth metatarsal heads (Frieberg's disease) and the lunate (Kienboch's disease) (*Figure 18.4*). Trauma appears to play some role in the aetiology of these conditions which may predispose to secondary osteoarthritis.

Pancreatic disease

Pancreatitis and pancreatic carcinoma may rarely cause disseminated fat necrosis. This may be followed by avascular necrosis or an arthritis. Subcutaneous fat necrosis gives rise to inflamed cutaneous nodules (ponniculitis) which are identical to erythema nodosum in appearance.

Pigmented villonodular synovitis

Most cases are young adults with painful swelling of a single knee. Other large joints are involved less frequently. There may be tenderness and swelling which is due to obvious synovial thickening.

Diagnostic suspicion may be aroused if aspirated joint effusion is blood-stained and there is no history of trauma. Radiographs may show subchondral cysts and loss of cartilage. Synovial biopsy often provides a firm diagnosis. The synovium tends to be brown, due to haemosiderin deposition, and villous formation is prolific. Histology reveals lining cell hyperplasia, a modest inflammatory cell infiltrate and many pigmented macrophages in the sub-synovium. The picture resembles that seen in haemophilia.

Synovectomy is the treatment of choice but since the synovium sometimes encroaches on soft tissue, as well as invading subchondral bone, radiotherapy may be used to supplement surgery.

Relapsing polychondritis

This disorder is rare and is one of widespread cartilage inflammation and necrosis. Pain in the nose and pinnae of the ears, arthritis and costal cartilage pain may reflect involvement of these sites. There may be insidious collapse of the nasal cartilage, giving rise to an appearance like a broken nose. The ears may become shrunken. Involvement and collapse of the tracheal rings may result in stridor and laryngeal inflammation causes hoarseness.

Other features may include iritis, aortic regurgitation, aneurysms and glomerulonephritis. Sometimes it is difficult to know whether these are part of the picture of polychondritis or an associated disease because it can occur in SLE, scleroderma and inflammatory bowel disease.

Corticosteroid treatment is helpful but treatment is often delayed because of difficulties with diagnosis. A 20% mortality occurs due principally to heart and tracheal involvement.

Sarcoidosis

Two patterns of sarcoid are recognized and both may be associated with arthritis. In the acute disease, erythema nodosum and hilar lymph node enlargement are accompanied by arthritis and peri-articular swelling, usually of the ankles and knees. The chronic disease may be associated with bone cysts which are apparent on radiographs of the fingers or toes. These are often related to the presence of cutaneous manifestations.

A chronic arthritis may involve large or small joints. This may cause erosions and is associated with the presence of sarcoid granulomata in the synovium.

Sickle cell disease

A compensatory expansion of bone marrow in homozygous disease produces a characteristic coarsening of trabeculae on radiographs. There may be thickening of the skull vault with a typical 'hair on end' appearance of the trabeculae. Vertebral bodies, softened by marrow encroachment of cancellous bone, may collapse, giving rise to a kyphosis.

Bone infarcts and avascular necrosis are acknowledged features. Less well recognized is a synovitis which may accompany crises. Effusions may occur but these tend to be non-inflammatory. The frequency of hyperuricaemia is increased.

Subacute bacterial endocarditis (SBE)

Arthralgia and a transient polyarthritis are features of a majority of patients with SBE. This may be immune complex-mediated, as is the cutaneous vasculitis seen in this disorder. Rarely, the arthritis may be due to infection within a joint cavity.

Synovial chondromatosis

Cartilage nodules form in the synovium of a large joint, usually the knee. These may calcify so that a radiograph may reveal multiple intra-articular opacities. The symptoms are those of a loose body within the joint with recurrent locking and effusions. Loose bodies may indeed be present as pieces of cartilage break free from the synovium. Synovectomy and removal of loose bodies is an effective treatment.

Urticaria

The rash of urticaria is pruritic and comprises a classical wheal. It may be seen as an allergic response to salicylates or other drugs and occurs in SLE, the prodrome of hepatitis B and as an isolated phenomenon (urticarial vasculitis). There may be arthralgia, proteinuria and peri-orbital or ankle oedema. It is a benign disorder when unassociated with any other illness. Progressive manifestations do not occur.

Further reading

CHURCHILL, M. *et al.* (1977). Musculoskeletal manifestations of bacterial endocarditis. *Ann. Intern. Med.*, **87,** 754

HOUGH, A. *et al.* (1976). Cartilage in hemophilic arthopathy. *Archs. Path.*, **100,** 91

JAMES, D. *et al.* (1976). Bone and joint sarcoidosis. Sem. *Arthritis Rheum.*, **6,** 53

KYLE, R. and BAYRD, E. (1975). Amyloidosis: review of 236 cases. *Medicine*, **54,** 271

MARTINEZLAVIN, M. *et al.* (1982). Hypertrophic osteoarthropathy in cyanotic congenital heart disease – its prevalence and relationship to bypass of the lung. *Arthritis Rheum.*, **25,** 1186

MOHSENIFAR, Z. *et al.* (1982). Pulmonary function in patients with relapsing polychondritis. *Chest*, **81,** 711

19
Anti-inflammatory and analgesic drugs

Medication for rheumatic diseases is heavily dependent on both non-steroidal anti-inflammatory drugs (NSAIDs) which have anti-inflammatory and analgesic properties and simple analgesic compounds which exert only an analgesic effect. In general, most rheumatic complaints have an inflammatory component which makes the NSAIDs a better option than simple analgesics. However, symptomatic control is often less than ideal with a NSAID and it is common practice to supplement treatment with an analgesic. This is more logical than combining anti-inflammatory drugs which are likely to have similar peripheral sites of action whereas analgesics usually have a central effect.

Non-steroidal anti-inflammatory drugs

The forerunner of these agents and the continuing yardstick by which newer drugs are measured is high dose aspirin. No NSAID has a more potent anti-inflammatory effect on joint inflammation than salicylates. However, the toxicity of salicylates, especially their propensity for causing gastric irritation and bleeding, have been the principal motivation for the development of better tolerated preparations. To some extent this has succeeded, but all NSAIDs share some of the undesirable effects of aspirin. A list of NSAIDs available in Britain is seen in *Table 19.1.*

TABLE 19.1 A list of most of the non-steroidal anti-inflammatory drugs currently available in Great Britain

Compound	Usual dose	Comments
Salicylates		
Soluble aspirin	1 g qds	Gastrointestinal side effects common
Aloxiprin	1 g qds	
Benorylate (aspirin/paracetamol)	2 g tds	Available as suspension
Choline magnesium trisalicylate	1.5 g bd	
Diflunisal	500 mg bd	Long half-life
Indoleacetic acids		
Indomethacin	25–50 mg tds	Useful in gout and ankylosing spondylitis. May cause headaches and other CNS effects
Sulindac	200–300 mg bd	A pro-drug
Tolectin	400 mg tds	Very short half-life
Phenylpropionic acids		
Ibuprofen	200–400 mg tds	Well tolerated
Fenoprofen	300–600 mg tds	–
Fenbufen	300–600 mg bd	A pro-drug
Ketoprofen	50 mg tds	–
Naproxen	500 mg bd	Long half-life
Tiaprofenic acid	200 mg tds	–
Pyrazolones		
Phenylbutazone	100 mg tds	Bone marrow toxicity. Useful for gout and ankylosing spondylitis but now available for the latter disease only
Azapropazone	600 mg bd	Uricosuric
Phenylacetic acids		
Diclofenac	50 mg tds	No interaction with anticoagulants
Fenamates		
Mefenamic acid	500 mg tds	Diarrhoea common
Oxicams		
Piroxicam	20 mg daily	Long half-life

Anti-inflammatory effects

An important, if not the major, property of NSAIDs is their inhibition of prostaglandin synthesis. Prostaglandins (PGs) have many important physiological functions amongst which is the mediation of inflammation (*see* Chapter 3). The NSAIDs may inhibit the cyclo-oxygenase pathway at one or several sites. None of the currently available drugs is known to have a major direct influence on the lipoxygenase pathway. There is experimental evidence to suggest that the anti-inflammatory action is not entirely dependent on PG inhibition. For example, in animals deficient in PG precursors, an anti-inflammatory effect can still be demonstrated.

Pharmacology

The NSAIDs are rapidly absorbed and most have a short half-life not exceeding 12 hours. A few have prolonged half-lives allowing once or twice daily dosage (fenbufen, piroxicam). Half-life may be increased by disease and ageing, especially if the drug undergoes metabolism before excretion.

Two agents, sulindac and fenbufen, are given as pro-drugs. Their activity is achieved only after hepatic metabolism. This lessens, but does not eliminate, the risk of gastric irritation.

All the NSAIDs are firmly bound to protein in the circulation. Activity is related to the free, unbound drug.

Side effects

A wide range of unwanted effects has been documented. These include nausea, vomiting, abdominal pain, diarrhoea, rashes, liver enzyme abnormalities and blurring of vision.

The gastrointestinal symptoms, especially those of the stomach, can be attributed to prostaglandin inhibition because PGE_2 protects the gut mucosa. Drugs given as enteric coated preparations, suppositories or pro-drugs reduce this effect in the gastric mucosa but not in the circulation. This explains why gastric side effects are so difficult to avoid.

The kidneys can be affected in several ways. Prostaglandins modulate renal blood flow and their inhibition reduces glomerular filtration. The NSAIDs can increase blood urea if renal function is already compromised but this is a reversible phenomenon. Renal PG inhibition may also explain the water and sodium retention occasionally seen. Interstitial nephritis or nephrotic syndrome are less common toxic manifestations. Analgesic abuse nephropathy due to renal papillary necrosis is more certainly caused by the analgesic phenacetin but salicylates are still viewed with suspicion.

It is well known that aspirin may induce asthma in susceptible subjects. It is less well appreciated that all NSAIDs may have the same effect. By blocking the cyclo-oxygenase pathway they cause a preferential increase of the lipoxygenase pathway and leukotriene activity. Some leukotrienes are bronchoconstrictors. The binding of NSAIDs to protein may displace concurrently prescribed anticoagulants and increase the risks of haemorrhage.

Simple analgesics

Non-narcotic drugs are preferable but are often inadequate treatment for chronic pain disorders. Paracetamol is the most useful of these but salicylates and other NSAIDs have analgesic properties in low doses.

The risk of addiction limits the value of narcotic analgesics but codeine phosphate, dihydrocodeine, dextropropoxyphene and dextropropoxyphene–paracetamol combinations are all of value. Nefopam is a relatively new analgesic with a central mode of action which is not known to be associated with risk of addiction.

Side effects commonly encountered with narcotic analgesics are nausea, vomiting and constipation.

Further reading

KANTOR, T. (1980). Analgesics for arthritis. *Clin. Rheum. Dis.*, **6,** 525
LIFSCHITZ, M. (1983). Renal effects of non-steroidal anti-inflammatory agents. *J. Lab. Clin. Med.*, **102,** 313

20
Role of the remedial professions

The medical and surgical treatments of rheumatic diseases are unable to eliminate disability. Resultant problems of function are often neglected or go unrecognized by doctors. Physiotherapists and occupational therapists have the expertise to provide an intimate assessment of the patient's physical difficulties and needs. They are also trained to encourage patients to achieve the optimal use of residual abilities. The skills of such personnel should be utilized to the full and their fund of knowledge exploited by both medical students and doctors.

Physiotherapists

The conventional aims of physiotherapy in rheumatic diseases are to:

1. reduce pain;
2. improve muscle power;
3. restore function; and
4. prevent or correct deformities.

Reduction of pain

The pain of inflammation may be reduced by rest in splints (*Figure 20.1*). These can be made from a range of materials, a task usually shared by occupational therapists.

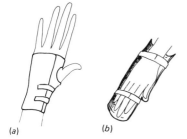

(a) (b)

Figure 20.1 Splints: (a) working splint for wrist; (b) resting splint for hand

Various physical treatments may be used to reduce pain. These include techniques for generating warmth, such as short wave diathermy and infrared lamps. Paradoxically, the application of ice is also used.

Other apparatus may interfere with perception or conduction of nerve pain impulses, e.g. interferential treatment or trans-cutaneous nerve stimulation. Laser and ultrasound are used to treat a wide range of painful disorders, especially of the soft tissues. Spinal pain is often treated by manipulation, traction or exercises.

Most of the above treatments are used empirically and have no proven therapeutic value beyond that of a placebo effect. This benefit should not be denied to patients for whom there are no other treatment options.

Improvement of muscle power

It is common for muscle wasting and weakness to develop rapidly in joint disease. Instruction and encouragement of sensible exercises may have a profound effect on the recovery or prevention of wasting. In painful and polyarticular disease, exercise can be facilitated by hydrotherapy. The buoyancy and soothing effect of warm water allows much greater freedom of movement.

Restoration of function

Reduction of pain and improved muscle power are measures which favour restoration of function. Advice about the importance of rest, posture, lifting, walking aids and transferring to and from bed or chair may need the emphasis of a therapist to achieve successful compliance. Most importantly, improvements of morale which may follow the involvement of a physiotherapist may have a dramatic influence on patients' capabilities.

Correction and prevention of deformities

The splinting of joints together with the use and preservation of surrounding muscles may limit deformities. Serial splints with a diminishing angle may correct developed deformities. Exercises and attention to posture may reduce stiffening deformity of the spine in ankylosing spondylitis.

Domiciliary physiotherapists may provide treatment at home. Hospital based therapists may profit from visiting patients' homes to determine their needs and treatment priorities.

Occupational therapists

The aims of the physiotherapist are shared by the occupational therapist who may be able to manufacture sophisticated resting or immobilizing splints, supervise muscle exercises orientated toward specific employment or domestic tasks and provide aids.

Assessment of patients' daily functions may be followed by training and practice in such functions as dressing, bathing and

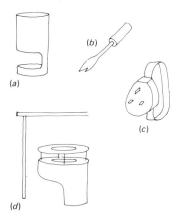

Figure 20.2 Aids for rheumatic patients: (a) light plastic beaker with recess for fingers; (b) fork-knife with thick rubber handle to aid grip; (c) electricity plug with handle for easy manipulation; (d) elevated lavatory seat and rail to help patients to stand from the sitting position

cooking. Aids may be necessary for some or all of these activities (*Figure 20.2*). The occupational therapist may be able to recommend either structural alterations to patients' homes, e.g. ramps and rails, or rehousing in more suitable accommodation. The ability to work may require assessment, and occupational therapists may provide retraining for new or previous employment. A knowlege of wheelchair designs makes occupational therapists ideally suited for recommending the appropriate model for individual patients.

The overlapping functions of therapists demand close liaision and this is often achieved by group discussions involving a doctor and other professional staff.

Appendix
Epidemiology of major rheumatic diseases

Disease	Incidence (No./population/year) or prevalance (%)	Peak age of onset	Sex distribution	Geographical or racial variations
Ankylosing spondylitis	0.4% adult males	20–30	M > F (4:1)	N. American Haida Indians > Caucasians > Negroes
Gout	0.4% adults	40–50	M > F (6:1)	(a) Affluent countries (b) Polynesians > Caucasians
Juvenile chronic arthritis	10/million children/year 0.06% school children	< 16	(a) Systemic M > F (b) Polyarticular F > M (c) Pauciarticular with (i) sacroiliitis M > F (ii) iridocyclitis F > M	
Osteoarthritis Radiological changes: (a) At any site (b) Hypertrophic, generalized	80% adults age > 55 15% F adults age > 44 10% M	> 50	F > M	Heberden nodes rare in Negroes

(c) Non-hypertrophic, generalized	8% F, 9% M } adults age > 44		F = M	
(d) Cervical spine	55% F, 78% M } adults age > 45		M > F	
(e) Lumbar spine	20% M, 13% F } all adults		M > F	
Polyarteritis nodosa	1/million/year	40–60	M > F (2:1)	
Polymyalgia rheumatica	300/million adults age > 70/year	> 60	F > M (2:1)	Caucasians > other races
Polymyositis/ dermatomyositis	2/million/year	40–60	F > M (2:1)	
Pseudogout Chondrocalcinosis	0.1% 25% adults age > 70	> 60	F = M	
Psoriatic arthritis	0.1%	35–45	F = M	
Reactive arthritis	1% patients with non-specific urethritis and 2% with *Shigella* infection	20–30	M > F	
Rheumatoid arthritis	1% adults	30–50	F > M (3:1)	Worldwide, all races
Scleroderma	2.7/million/year	30–50	F > M (5:1)	
Systemic lupus erythematosus	0.04% (USA)	20–40	F > M (9:1)	Negroes > Asians > Caucasians

Index

Achilles tendonitis, 179
Acromegaly, 29, 64, 177, 183
Acute arthritis, 107–130
Acute phase proteins, 24
Adhesive capsulitis, 173, 174
  in diabetes, 182
Agammaglobulinaemia, 185
Alcohol,
  and hyperuricaemia, 113
  effects of, 185
  liver disease and, 191
Algodystrophy, 185
Alkaptonuria, 29, 183
Allergic granulomatous vasculitis, 159
Amyloid A, 39
Amyloid nephropathy, 39, 50
Amyloidosis, 86, 186
Amyloid P component, 39
Anaemia,
  in ankylosing spondylitis, 82
  in juvenile chronic arthritis, 165
  in polymyalgia rheumatica, 104
  in psoriatic arthropathy, 89
  in rheumatoid arthritis, 39
  sickle cell, 194
Analgesics, 199
Ankles,
  in Behçet's syndrome, 99
  in rheumatoid arthritis, 35
  osteoarthritis of, 27
Ankylosing spondylitis, 53, 76–86, 96
  aetiology, 83
  children and, 166
  course of, 86
  diagnosis and investigations, 58, 82
  epidemiology, 204

Ankylosing spondylitis (cont.)
  pathology of, 84
  symptoms and signs, 80
  Tietze's syndrome in, 178
  treatment, 85
Ankylosis, in rheumatoid arthritis, 40
Annulus fibrosus, 3
Antibodies,
  anti-Sm, 22
  anti-RNP, 22
  identification, 22
  Ro, 22
Antibody-dependent cellular
  cytotoxicity, 15, 42
Anti-cardolipin antibodies, 137
Anticentromere antibody, 145
Antigens,
  phagocytosis, 14
  processing, 2
Antigen-antibody complexes, 21
Anti-inflammatory drugs, 196
  See also specific compounds
  effects, 197
  non-steroidal, 196
  pharmacology, 198
  side effects, 198
Antinuclear antibodies, 21
Antinuclear factor, in systemic lupus
  erythematosus, 135
Aortic disease,
  in ankylosing spondylitis, 81, 85
  in polymyalgia rheumatica, 106
Arachnoiditis, 63
Arboviruses, 130
Arthritis,
  acute, 107–130

207

215